Caregiving: How to Survive And Get Out Alive.

Things I've Figured Out After A Decade of Caregiving.

Joy Walker

Dedicated to Sue Gammicchia, the first caregiver I ever knew, and to Ross, mentor and friend, who helped show me what I could do.

Table of Contents

***

Acknowledgments.

I would like, first and always, to thank Jill for being my sounding board, my friend, and my biggest cheerleader, for helping me to stay mobile and physically able to write, and for helping me navigate through the rocky shoals of life. For Paul, who loves me and fights hard. To my dear friend Alex, who always listens, and Theresa and Steve – thanks for being my family. Erica, my "lovely and amazing friend" who is just starting this journey, and is doing an exemplary job – thank you for letting me put you in the book. Big thanks go to Greg, Marica and the wonderful staff at Marica's AFH for truly loving Dad and wanting the best for him.

I want to thank the good people at Providence Hospice, especially Wendi, who trusted me to know how to hold space in a group of grieving people and helped me grow. This book is for all the incredible people at the LBDA, who work tirelessly, many of them unpaid, to support caregivers and spread the word about Lewy body dementia. It is also for my support group members, who taught me so much and who have humbled me with their stories, and for caregivers everywhere, who are going above and beyond every single day of their lives.

Author's Notes

In order to protect privacy, some of the names and identifying characteristics have been changed, and in some cases I have made composites of several individuals and/or cases. I've preserved the chronology of events as well as I could, but have made some changes for the sake of narrative flow or discretion. Those changes aside, these are true events and this is a true story, constructed from memory.

30% of the proceeds from sale of the book will be donated to the LBDA.

1.

It's About the Journey.

"Our deepest calling is to grow into our own authentic self-hood, whether or not it conforms to some image of who we ought to be. As we do so, we will not only find the joy that every human being seeks -- we will also find our path of authentic service in the world." Parker J. Palmer

I realized the other day, after looking at a calendar, that I have been my father's caregiver for more than ten years now, which is a long time by anybody's standards. If I had given birth, I would now be the parent of a ten year old. Instead, I have watched the process go in reverse, and seen my father become infantilized. More has happened in these ten years than I could have imagined. They have been the best, and perhaps the hardest, years of my life. They have certainly involved the most changes.

When you are a caregiver – whether young or old, male or female, spouse or adult child or even parent – you learn pretty quickly that things rarely stay the same from day to day. What worked one day doesn't the next, what was a definite symptom one week disappears the next, what you need one month changes the next. Expect the best, prepare for the worst becomes every caregiver's motto. Every day is a little different.

Eleven years ago, when I became Dad's caregiver, I was actually accustomed to this truism. Living with a chronic illness, rheumatoid arthritis, means that life can change day to day. You get used to daily changes in how you feel, what your body is doing, and what you're able to do that particular day. Maybe that's why I was able to adjust more easily than some caregivers to Dad's behavior and symptoms changing weekly – along with his needs. As dementia progresses, all caregivers struggle to keep up with their loved ones' care, and behaviors, and healthcare and housing needs. Flexibility becomes paramount, which can be tough if you're already tired and at the end of your rope and have been giving care for years and years.

Like many caregivers, I had to assume a role I neither trained for nor expected to have to perform and I had to learn how to do it while on the job. For many years before his dementia, my father and I had a complex relationship, defined mostly by the distances between us – physically, emotionally, and ideologically. Late in 2003, after years of denial that there was anything really wrong with my father, I discovered his dementia had progressed past the point where he was safe living by himself. I became a caregiver.

Suddenly, our lives were attached – conjoined. Adjustments had to be made, re-evaluations were required, balances shifted, and a lot of therapy undertaken. I obtained full time, twenty-four hour care for him, allowing him to remain at home. I also began the torturous, tedious process of learning how to manage someone else's finances, health care, housing, and legal affairs.

The first five years of being Dad's caregiver were fairly tumultuous. We experienced a lot of change and challenge together, much of which I wrote about in my first book – a memoir about my first three years caregiving and the six months I spent cleaning out his house. It's been difficult, and a struggle, and absolutely maddening – and at the very same time, it's been funny, deepening, and enlightening – and we've lived it together. Years ago, our stories became a story, one that never ceases to surprise me.

*

This is my story – a story about eleven years, and counting, in the life of a young(ish) caregiver. It is the story of me, my dad, and his dementia. This is the story of the people who have shared my caregiving journey with me and the wonderful, terrible, challenging and amazing events and experiences that have made up my life as a caregiver and a woman, so far. I am sometimes surprised at the twists and turns this story has taken, and I wonder how many more it will take before it is over. It sometimes feels like I've lived a whole lifetime in just the last four years, let alone the last eleven.

Trying to have any kind of life while being a caregiver for someone with dementia is like walking on a floor covered with marbles – you can do it but it takes a lot of concentration, a willingness to go in random directions, and the ability to get back up repeatedly. I have had the feet pulled out from under me more times than I'm really happy about, and I've ended up in different places than I originally intended. But I have continued to have my own life while being a caregiver; fitting in dating and relationships, illnesses and recoveries, and personal and professional transformations.

Dad's illness, though sad, was the genesis of many good things, including a better relationship between us, although it was also difficult to see him deteriorate. There were other big emotional changes, as well, primarily in my personal life. I learned that I could survive, and actually thrive, as a caregiver – that I could have my own life even while caring for Dad's. I embarked on a serious romantic relationship, had a minor career as a multi-media artist, traveled, wrote the memoir, and started a blog. And that was just in the first five years of being a caregiver!

In these last five years, after some adjustments to Dad's care and living situation, things have settled down in terms of his illness and needs. He seems to be in something of a lull, his illness progressing slowly – the half-time break before the difficult last part of a long and stressful game. Being in this relative lull of Dad activity has opened up space for more surprising changes in my personal and professional/spiritual life.

It has allowed me the time to find out as much as I could about the different types of dementia, explore the difficult undertaking that is caregiving, and attain some training that might help me help other caregivers. It has given me the chance to find an environment in which I can use the random and various skills, strengths, and knowledge that I have collected over the years to serve others and make a difference, as well as giving me the chance to try to build a life to support myself after Dad dies – an event I know is coming.

I ended the first romantic relationship and embarked on another one – even getting married. I won awards for my blog and began writing for other blogs, websites, and publications. I traveled abroad and studied how other countries are approaching the problems of dementia and caregivers. And I founded, and facilitate for, two dementia support groups. In short, I grew, more than I had ever expected.

Although most caregivers would probably say it's impossible to live your own life while giving care, I am here to say that it is not impossible but it requires an openness to what is coming next, a desire to continue to live and experience life, and a certainty that one's life is worth as much as one's care receiver. I want to tell other caregivers that you can survive – and thrive – even while giving care. I want to tell them that it is, in fact, absolutely necessary to have some sort of life of one's own – both to make the duties of caregiving easier, but also to have something to turn to when caregiving is done. That their lives matter just as much as the lives of their loved one, and that they deserve their space on this earth.

*

This is the story of all caregivers, whose experiences are all different and unique, and yet they share so many commonalities and similarities; enough so that telling just one story can often help many. After enough counseling and talking to other caregivers and pondering my own experiences, I recognized that, although everyone's experience is decidedly different from everyone else's, there were a few main struggles and shibboleths of caregiving that always seemed to be present, to emerge in conversation, to be "up."

I wanted to collect these issues in one place, out in the open, where they could be discussed plainly, and where people could feel they were not alone in their experiences of them – kind of like one of my support groups! I feel like I have better ideas now about what needs to be talked about and about what caregivers need to hear. So, I wrote a second book, covering the whole ten years of my experience, so that I could share those ideas, as well as new information and support with as many other caregivers as possible.

As most caregivers can attest to, the minute a diagnosis is confirmed, everything changes, and will keep changing, sometimes daily, until the end. Dementia and the need for caregiving transforms life, usually in challenging and uncomfortable ways. I know that it can sometimes seem to caregivers as if there have only ever been negative changes, never positive, and that nothing good will ever happen again. I want them to know that others share their pain and confusion and absolute frustration with disappearing family members, uncaring physicians, and financial and bureaucratic labyrinths.

There are others that understand the difficulties inherent in fighting through denial, learning about illness, and taking your loved one's car keys. Others who have had to learn to connive and lie and make things work the best they can. Others who have had to move loved ones who haven't wanted to be moved, and dealt with the ensuing guilt and emotional blackmail. There are others who have survived caregiving, which means that if they can – anyone can.

I have written about my experiences, and the experiences of many of the people I talk to, in an effort to spread that work and possibly introduce new ways of thinking to whoever needs it. These stories are for all of these people, and all the people who will soon be joining us among the ranks of caregiver. Those who read my first book (and thank you, by the way) may recognize some of the stories I use as examples.

I used these stories again because I am looking at them now through the lens of my experience and training, and my exposure to other caregivers – exposure I did not yet have when I wrote the first book. I wanted to integrate these past events with everything new that has occurred and make something different that will, hopefully, resonate with other caregivers.

In revisiting all of the events of Dad's illness so far, I see where I stumbled and where I excelled. I see the mistakes I made and how my choices played out. I see where I would have done so much better – felt so much better – if I had possessed different, or more, information. All of these things are what I share with people and other caregivers every day, spreading the word about how to give care more effectively and live your own life, too – something I believe with all my heart is possible to do. Just remember that every day is going to be a little different, and you'll do just fine.

*

I have included short, pithy takeaways at the end of each caregiving chapter detailing what I've figured out after more than a decade of giving care, with quick information to help those who don't have time to read the whole chapter. So read the book however you need to – back to front, front to back, or only the tips at the end.

In addition, I have found that most of the terms that describe those who are receiving care are neither graceful nor precise. I have used and known others to use: "charge", "caree", "care receiver", "care partner", and "loved one." Nobody can seem to come to an agreement about which word is best, and we all tend to use them interchangeably. I have settled on "care receiver" as the most clear.

2.

Denial – Not Just a River in Egypt.

"The thing about denial is that it doesn't feel like denial when it's going on."
Georgina Kleege.

My father could fix anything; the list of things he had repaired just in my lifetime was enormous. I believed I could rely on him to know how to deal with any project, so I naturally called him for help the day the ceramic soap dish attached to the wall in my shower fell off. I suspected we would need some sort of adhesive or caulking but that he would know exactly what was required and would be able to fix it quickly.

When we walked into Home Depot, looking for the right tools and materials, I was shocked when he didn't seem to know what we needed. "I thought YOU knew what we were getting!" he said with a laugh and a somewhat sheepish expression, when I asked repeatedly what type of caulk or glue we might need to use. We eventually managed to pick out a product and reattach the soap dish, but we both knew something bad had happened, we just weren't sure what, or how to handle it.

Over the next five years, I started to see more strange behaviors from my father but, like many others before me, I resolutely turned my head, averted my eyes, and didn't want to know about it. It started out so small, as these things so often do - little occurrences that you could almost convince yourself were nothing. Like the afternoon he was supposed to drive over to my house, only twenty minutes or so away from his. I waited and waited but he didn't arrive, and when I finally phoned him, angry that he had blown me off, he was apologetic and seemed shaken. He said that he had felt too nervous to try to drive the route, which was shocking, considering these were roads he'd been driving since I was born.

My dad loved cars and he loved driving and I began to realize that he didn't seem to be driving nearly as much as in the past. He insisted he just didn't feel like going out as much, and we never talked about it again. Several times, we made appointments to meet at my house or somewhere else and he wouldn't show up, claiming when I called that he had completely forgotten that we had arranged anything, sounding lost and bewildered.

I knew deep down, of course, what was probably going on – after all, everybody knows what cognitive problems look like - but I found it impossible to relate it to my father. I wasn't prepared to even admit there might be a problem to myself, let alone talk to him about it.

He called me one day asking for my help with some banking correspondence that he couldn't make sense of, asking if I would come see him and help him figure out what was needed. The phone call alone was shocking since he was famously paranoid about his money and banking details, and to admit that he needed help in that area was unprecedented. When I arrived at his house, ready to help, he was delighted to see me but obviously didn't remember that we had made the date. I was shocked, it was one of the biggest and most noticeable cognitive failures that I had witnessed with him, and I knew in my heart that things were bad. I wasn't sure they were going to get better, and was pretty sure they were only going to get worse.

When I gently reminded him that *he* had called *me* about a problem, I could see his face crumple with the recognition that something was terribly, terribly wrong, but he just couldn't face it.

The closest he got to admitting he knew something wasn't right was the fact that tears filled his eyes while he put an arm around me and apologized quietly for wasting my time. Neither one of us were prepared to put a name to what we had just experienced, however, I know what I was thinking – Alzheimer's.

*

The first call from the police went to my sister, requesting that she come to a local elementary school to pick up our Father, who had been found wandering cold and confused on the playground, located about five miles from his home. We had known of his penchant for long (really long), healthy walks, but had been unaware that he was starting to forget how to get *home* from them. Upon taking him home, we finally got a good look at his home and realized that there was more going on with him than just getting a little disoriented on a walk. Something else was seriously wrong.

The house was cold, dank, and filled with mildew due to the fact that the furnace was broken and he was relying on the fireplace and one space heater for warmth. In addition, he had become something of a hoarder, saving every slip of paper and junk mail, newspaper, and plastic container and soda bottle that came into the house. It looked like a trash heap. We also discovered that he had been eating very poorly, when he ate at all. He seemed primarily to be consuming carbohydrates like bread, crackers, chips, cookies, and potato salad, with some cans of beans and franks thrown in. He also seemed to be drinking mostly soda, if the number of empty cleaned out bottles was anything to go by. He was painfully thin, was obviously not doing laundry, and was dressed in multiple layers of clothing in an effort to stay warm, which hid his thinness.

Dad had always struggled with depression but it seemed like his mental state had gotten completely out of hand and he was living almost like a homeless person. Writing about this now, it seems both shameful and shocking that we had so little idea about what was going on, however, I have to remember that neither one of us were regular visitors to my dad's house since we each had our own difficult relationship with him.

My mother died in 1990, and since she was the glue that held our family together, it became harder to stay in touch. I usually felt responsible for him, so would call every few weeks or invite him to dinner. When he and I went out to eat, I usually picked him up in his driveway or we met somewhere. Since I didn't visit the house very often, not liking to be there without my mom, I was unaware of the extent to which it had disintegrated.

Before we left him, we made plans to all meet in his home a few days later to discuss the problem. When my sister and I got there, the house was cold, dark, and empty, so we waited in her car in the driveway for an hour before watching as a strange car drove up to the house and dropped my father off. I approached the car and spoke to the driver to determine what was going on. Apparently, he had become disoriented once again on the walk home and been picked up by this kind woman; somehow, he was able to convey to her his address and she brought him home.

After we hustled him into the house, my sister and I were appalled and attempted to communicate our shock at the situation to my father, who, as I remember, was uncooperative. He tried to brush off our concerns by breaking down each point we made into its basic components and refuting each one – a tactic other caregivers will be familiar with. He had an answer for each problem, a reason for each scary event, an excuse for each failure of decision making and self-care. He was too busy to do laundry or eat; didn't want to spend the money on a new furnace; was making the much-needed house repairs himself, but in his own time; had just gotten tired and forgotten a few directions in the dark; thought that the police were intrusive and trying to take control of his life. Excuse after excuse – it was impossible to battle them all.

Neither my sister nor I knew anything about caregiving – or dementia. We could tell that something was really wrong just from his behavior, his forgetfulness, and the increasingly parlous state of his house and living conditions but were at a loss as to what to do. We were also in the process of dealing with our own lives, and I had the added pressure of a chronic illness to manage. Neither one of us wanted to expend the sizeable emotional and physical energy it would take to battle through Dad's paranoia, secrecy, and subterfuge and get him to start talking about the problem.

We knew that my father should probably not be living alone, however, neither one of us were willing or able to move in with him. It was doubtful he would agree to some hired aide living in the house, and how were we supposed to go about finding one? It was even more doubtful that he would agree to go to a facility.

I know now that we ignored far too many warning signs, and we waited too long to step in, putting Dad's well-being in danger. We were also putting others' well-being in danger since he was still driving periodically – and unsafely. If I had it to do again, I would do it all differently, but I guess you can only do the best you can according to what you know to do. We were facing problems we had never imagined we would face and being forced to fight through patterns of denial laid down from childhood.

*

I know a lot about denial because my family was perfect in every way. Or at least, we were perfectly good at being in denial, the roots of which stretched far back into my parents' past. I know so little about their childhood– I only have snippets of information, and anecdotes, and family myth that I have pieced together and used to explain their later lives and existence as parents.

I know very little about my father's father, Arthur, and not much more about my grandmother, Mildred. I think Art struggled with his responsibilities to his family, and I believe he moved them around a lot in search of the perfect job. I know that at one point, they lived on a farm in Florida; later, my grandfather would own a combination bicycle/tool/parts shop, although it is my understanding that he was a very poor businessman.

I believe my grandmother had been something of a tomboy as a girl, growing up into an intelligent, independent, and acerbic woman. She was a writer and a teacher, at one point even writing a memoir about her experiences teaching low income kids in Detroit, Michigan. I don't think she was a particularly warm or affectionate woman – she certainly wasn't by the time I met her. I believe she was a spiritual person, although I know that she regularly switched religions between Protestant Christianity and Christian Science.

My father was the oldest of four children – two girls and two boys. He grew up sailing, working, and fiddling with anything technological or mechanical he could get his hands on; including radios, televisions, and vehicles. My dad could fix or build anything mechanical – he was gifted with an engineer's mind, and attended a technical high school.

I believe that they were living in Michigan when my father's brother, upon hitting puberty, began to exhibit strange and anti-social behaviors. My grandmother knew there was something seriously wrong with her son, but it appears that she had a difficult time convincing her husband or other children to admit it or get involved. This is one of the first serious occurrences of denial that I know of in my family. My uncle would eventually be diagnosed with Schizophrenia, but it was the white elephant in the family – apparently nobody really wanted to talk about it.

It was around this time that my grandfather began to yearn to move back to Florida to open his bike/parts/tool shop, and my grandmother, struggling with my sick uncle and her other young children, refused to uproot the family and move. My grandfather left anyway, and they eventually divorced. Perhaps it was this train of events that caused my grandmother to begin a lifelong dedication to women's liberation and women's rights, and I also believe she took her anger at my grandfather, and all men, out on my father. I think all of these events marked a turning point of shock and stress for my father.

Abandonment by his father during a critical stage of adolescence; his mother's retreat into anger, resentment, and hypercritical behavior, likely paired with an increased dependence on her son - my father; and the out-of-nowhere illness of his brother, showing him that the body and mind can betray one at any time. I believe that it was perhaps at this time that he subconsciously made several decisions about how things worked and how he wanted his life to be.

I think my father was so scared about his brother's illness and the capriciousness of the human system that he began to follow in my grandmother's religious footsteps as a Christian Scientist. He was much more fervent, however, in his beliefs, whereas she would probably have been more relaxed in her faith. I think my father feared that he had the same seeds of mental illness in himself as his brother, and was finding any tool he could against it.

I do know that he attended MIT for his freshman year of college and that he didn't return, either because of money or because he flunked out. I believe it was the latter. He would eventually complete his bachelors and masters degrees in electrical engineering at Wayne State University, but perhaps it was this failure at MIT that also sparked some of the fear, depression, and semi-withdrawal from life that would come later.

I don't know, exactly, when my father's battles with depression began – in young adulthood, after his failure at college? The "black moods", as we called them, were a part of life from my earliest memory. During these dark times, my father would stalk around the house glowering and angry. These episodes could last for weeks – weeks of grouchy trips to and from work, a morose face and monosyllabic responses at the dinner table, and as little interaction with his family as possible. And then suddenly, he would be better, approachable, and relatively happy.

He was never manic – or at least I don't remember that he was – he would just seem to snap out of it, and would start to interact with us again and act like a dad, until it happened again. From a young age and with a child's self-centered world view, I remember wondering what I had done to make him so angry. As I got older, I remember wondering why nobody talked about it, why nobody addressed at the dinner table the huge white elephant of my father's mood – but nobody did, instead, we compared notes as to who had done what that might have pissed him off. It seemed a little odd that he would withdraw himself from us so completely for so long, but I never really compared it to the behavior of my friends' fathers, and it just became normal.

I have about the same amount of information about my mother. She remains an almost shadowy figure, insubstantial and half-remembered. I have only childish perceptions, two dimensional and probably imprecise, memories, and impressions tainted by my adult thoughts. I must sift through these things now as an adult, trying to make sense of them, trying to place myself in that child space again to determine whether what I *remember* thinking or concluding as a child is what actually happened, or has just been influenced by who I am today.

My mother was the only child of older parents, who were actually surprised (and as family legend has it – unhappy) when they learned they were pregnant. Regardless of their feelings at first, after my mother was born, she became the apple of their eye. By the time my mother arrived, my grandparent's relationship had already broken down into a mixture of dependency, enmity, and fondness that I would witness years later. My grandmother was a devout Christian Scientist, and my mother followed her into the religion, albeit without the same strong beliefs.

My grandfather was an alcoholic and I know it had a negative effect on my mother. She carried a lot of repressed anger and resentment, feelings I now know to be common in children of alcoholics. Although she was both pretty and smart – winning a scholarship to college due to her grades and attitude, being one example – I don't believe she had very much self-esteem or belief in herself. She ended up not taking the scholarship, instead becoming a secretary at nineteen, when she met my twenty-four year old father at a Christian Science social mixer. They married a year later. It was the shared background in Christian Science that brought them together - a religion which would foster and enhance their inclinations toward denial of their mental and emotional states, as well as their physical and emotional needs, and those of their daughters.

My mother was definitely our primary nurturer and confidante, and I have no doubt that she loved us dearly. She was also deeply angry, however; at her alcoholic father; at her depressed and often disconnected husband; and, I think, at her sense of disappointment about her life. This anger manifested in many different ways, directed both at herself and at my sister and I, but never directly at my father.

She suffered from an eating disorder and was always on some sort of diet, while at the same time loving food and how it made her feel. She would become wildly angry and would lose her temper, swearing and slamming cupboard, car, and oven doors – sometimes breaking things in her rage. She was also engaged in an odd, and silent, campaign against my father, enlisting us as part of her special club, and emotionally separating us from him. We would do fun events during the day which she would then instruct us not to talk about so that we didn't "hurt his feelings", or make him mad that we were having fun without him. I felt sorry for, and probably responsible for, my father's isolation and struggled to connect with him and make him feel loved and part of the family, even while I was a part of my mother's "club."

My parents discouraged open discussion of our thoughts and emotions, silently encouraging us to deal with our problems independently, from a very young age. We were actively discouraged from expressing ourselves emotionally. It was understood early on by my sister and I that it was best to keep most of our emotions to ourselves – in fact, it was best if emotions or contrary opinions didn't exist at all.

I would no sooner have broached the subject of my father's depression and isolation or my mom's deep rage and lack of voice then I would have considered flying, although, admittedly, I often *thought* about doing it. Composing these sentences and arguments in my head led to a lifelong tendency to plan out whatever I want to say, refining it several times before it leaves my mouth.

My sibling and I were expected to be mature, self-sufficient, and emotionally stable. On the surface, we were an average family – close-knit, living a good life in the suburbs in a nice house, taking family vacations, working and playing. I know this is something you could say about a million families: that nothing is ever what it seems, that parents can be stern or difficult or neglectful, and that there are hidden dysfunctions and even some denial. But the thing that caused my family to positively *steep* in denial was the Christian Science.

*

Christian Science depends on the belief that everything is actually a perfect reflection of God, and any dysfunction or problem that manifests is a deviation from this truth. Your body (and the entire material world around you) is an illusion. Christian Scientists deny most of the realities of the human body and the physical world. They don't believe in illness, death, or medical intervention, instead depending on prayer for healing and guidance.

It is a religion based on words: passages read in rote repetition from the Bible, and from the Christian Science text book, *Science and Health with Key to the Scriptures,* which was written by the founder, Mary Baker Eddy, supposedly as a direct missive from God. Their doctrine asserts that disease and dysfunction are solely the result of negative thoughts and belief systems; that prayer and repetition of certain texts can cure disease; and that medication and medical intervention was unnecessary.

Of course, Christian Science suited my father's naturally ascetic and stoical nature. During one memorable occasion, he broke his right wrist skiing, yet refused to get it attended to. He continued on in the face of pain and discomfort, using his left hand to shift gears when driving and to write. At some point, however, the discomfort must have defeated him and he came home with a cast, which no one in our house ever mentioned. He seemed to prefer to believe that he could control all of his body's needs and actions – keep them under control like puppies on a tight leash. Christian Science's program of self-abnegation suited him perfectly.

My mother followed my father's lead, however, she would never be as devout as he was and we always knew somehow that she wasn't as convinced. Reading some of her correspondence many years later, I learned that these doubts troubled her and made her feel shallow and fickle. She would never know that her doubts would be our salvation - the loophole through which my sister and I could believe that if there was something seriously wrong with us, she might be able to help.

Almost from the beginning, my sister and I would believe as she did. However, we still trotted obediently off to church as a family every Sunday morning to go to Sunday school to be indoctrinated into the belief system.

We were taught that if we read repetitive passages and prayers out of the Bible and the *Science and Health*, and truly believed them, that we would be absolutely fine. I did try to absorb these concepts into my mind, but they were very difficult for a child to understand. As children, my sister and I were routinely shamed when we were ill or hurt. Any discussion of our bodies or physical issues was frowned upon, and we were encouraged to pray for ourselves when we suffered an injury or illness.

As with so many other things in my family, we had a sort of second life when we were sick that my mother tried to keep from my dad – more denial. It was our little secret. If we had a moderate illness, like a cold or upset stomach, we could stay home on the couch, but we were cleaned up before my dad got home along with all trace of illness – a charade he pretended to believe.

If we were very ill, with a fever or infection of some sort, we might be allowed to stay on the couch, but would feel the weight of our dad's disapproval that we had succumbed to erroneous thought. If we were really lucky, he might come over and sit with us and share some passages of the *Science and Health*, during which he abjured us to turn our thoughts towards right thinking, away from believing we had an illness, towards prayer and the Bible.

He was actually asking us to participate in some pretty grown-up philosophies and beliefs, and I know we struggled to please him. It left us feeling ashamed and guilty every time we felt sick, made it impossible to ask for help or believe our needs were valid or important, and left us deeply uncertain that we would receive much assistance, even from our mother, if anything serious were to happen to us. We were lucky enough to avoid any serious problems as children, however, the effects of Christian Science would be harmful and long-reaching for the entire family and would end up causing serious and long-term physical and emotional consequences for both me and my sister.

In keeping with the family's tendency towards denial, after my mother found a lump in her breast, she waited until her breast was misshapen before finally getting it checked. Interestingly, after the diagnosis, she went straight to Western medicine: I have no idea what conversations she and my father may have had, nor what pressure he may have applied on her, if any, to use Christian Science. She had her breast removed, along with many lymph nodes, and had chemotherapy, and radiation, as well as reconstructive surgery.

After two years, she suffered an occurrence of skin cancer on her chest from the radiation; a fact she kept from my sister and me, only telling my father. Three years after that, on the late-September weekend my parents moved me into the dorm for my first year of college, I noticed that she had a bad cough and seemed tired. In November, she would call me with a diagnosis of lung cancer; by July, she would be actively dying. By the first week of August, she would be dead. As a family, we hardly spoke about it, before or after her death.

All of her clothes stayed in her closet for years, along with scarves and handbags and shoes. Underwear and socks stayed in dresser drawers, books and treasured knick-knacks stayed on shelves. Furniture, even the couch my mom died on, stayed put, getting older and older. The house, and my father, just seemed to keep gently disintegrating. We rarely spoke about my mother, never talked about her cancer, and I acknowledged the anniversary of her death privately each year. After many years, Dad moved her clothes downstairs to the closet in a spare room. Eventually, I got rid of them when I was cleaning out the house. It was not as if he couldn't accept that she had died – he knew she was dead - it was that he was so good at not thinking about anything he didn't want to think about.

Dad was a Master at denial, and we were his pupils, which was what made it so difficult to go against our training when his situation became serious. It was so much easier to shut our eyes and our ears to the problem. I'm not sure if we hoped that it would improve on its own, or that something would come along that took care of it for us.

*

I tell the story about denying Dad's **evident** illness, even though it makes me look bad, because I want people to know I understand the siren song of denial. I know how deeply family rules and accepted behaviors can go and I know how difficult it can be to circumvent them when something serious happens. I know that even when you *think* you've seen the situation clearly and are taking some sort of action, you can still be in denial: you can still be expecting something that isn't going to happen, or hoping for an improvement or a change that's not coming, or seeing a person that is no longer there.

Whatever your family history and experience, everyone has faced denial. I have heard so many denial stories, from strangers, friends, and the people I've talked to. It is an across-the-board reaction – Elizabeth Kubler-Ross included it into her Grief cycle for a reason. A little bit of denial is actually a natural, healthy response. It is a way for the mind to make some space around new facts, giving us the time and capacity to accept and absorb new realities.

Facing change is never an easy thing to accept and there will inevitably be some reluctance to acknowledge it.

Denial is an established step on the long road that is caregiving. It is part of the process, happening at the beginning, the middle, and the end. It happens to the person needing care, you, the potential caregiver, and to the family. The illness of a family member will never be a clear and simple matter, with clear and simple choices. Illness and change are rocks thrown into a calm pond, causing ripple effects to radiate out from the point of impact, disturbing the peace of the water, affecting not just the care-taker but those around them.

It is, understandably, hard for anyone to believe that either they themselves or a loved one could be ill, or failing, or anything other than the capable, competent, ever-present adult they've always been. I know this to be true in my experiences with my illness. Even though I accepted the physical fact of having an illness – visiting the doctor, taking my medications, arranging my schedule to accommodate my fatigue and diminished physical capacity – *emotionally*, I was in denial. I pushed myself too hard, did too much, and allowed a lot of physical stress to my body that I shouldn't have. All because I didn't want to fully admit to myself that I had a condition I would be dealing with for the rest of my life – a condition that limited me.

A diagnosis of a long-term illness like rheumatoid arthritis or lupus or cancer with its attendant pain and suffering or of dementia coupled with the contemplation of years and years of horror, humiliation, and heartbreak is not what any of us want to hear.

Denial can provide that comfortable emotional space for everyone to inhabit as it precludes immediately accepting unpleasant truths and the necessity to take action. Let's face it, any illness in a loved one would be tough to accept.

When trying to understand why it's so hard to fight denial in oneself, and admit that something is not right with a loved one, don't underestimate your fear. Fear of losing that person, fear of what will happen to them, and fear of the huge ways your life will change, because they will be huge. Denial has its roots in fear: fear of loss; fear of pain and suffering; fear of confrontation and emotions and fear of the future and the ways we and our loved ones will change.

I was immobilized by the fears of what my father having dementia would mean to me. At first, I was too sick and tired to want to act, and then I was too happy with where my life was heading to contemplate the huge earthquake that was my father's potential dementia. I'm not proud when I say that I have no idea how far I would have let things go if Dad's wandering, and the Mercer Island police, hadn't decided the issue for me! Accepting my father's dementia required all the things I was afraid of: rearranging and adding a burden to my own life; discussing unpleasant truths with my ill Father, convincing him that he needed to give up years of life and independence; and breaking through everyone else's denial process as much as possible so that we could all be happy and safe.

So many people report having seen worrying signs of dysfunction long before a crisis, and are subsequently angry with themselves for allowing matters to reach critical mass before stepping in. I can only tell them my own experience and that it was solely by the grace of God that nothing too damaging happened. This is not easy stuff. Perhaps you've started seeing the same kind of things that I did - maybe worse, maybe better - but you haven't yet acted on it. One of my worst moments was discovering that my father had been eating so poorly - it was unclear whether he got any proteins or vegetables – and living so roughly and uncomfortably.

Maybe you've noticed your loved one isn't as well-groomed and dressed as usual, or that they are forgetting basic tasks like going out for groceries, paying bills, or feeding themselves. Maybe you've noticed that cognitively, your loved one is still lucid, but they are staying at home more, not doing favorite past-times. Maybe they just don't seem well. There are lots of resources now that tell individuals what signs to look for, but that still doesn't make it any easier to take that first step. You will always question what you are seeing and feeling.

Sometimes a situation progresses slowly, like ours, making it easy to ignore or put off what needs to be done. Sometimes, the health of a loved one can change in as little as a few days, a week, or a month, causing a crisis - since nobody is prepared for it, it can be difficult to accept and adjust quickly. We'd rather play it safe, believe in a comfortable lie for as long as possible, than have to deal with painful reality.

Whether a situation unfolds over time or becomes urgent quite quickly, different members of the family will respond differently, adjusting in their own ways to a painful new reality. I hear from caregivers who are actively impeded by parents, aunts, uncles, and other family members who either haven't seen the problem first hand, or don't believe in it. I tell these caregivers to have that family member come over for a few hours or days so that they can see the reality for themselves. Sometimes caregivers may experience a complete disappearance of their loved one's good friends, hurting and disappointing both care receiver and caregiver. Friends may be in denial out of fear of being near the disease, or grief at the potential loss of a friend.

You will never get me to say that it was anything but agonizingly difficult and a huge challenge to trump my excellent training in denial. It is why I empathize so much with new caregivers who have so much to fight through before they can get down to what needs doing. Everything did work out, more or less, for the best, however. I do believe that putting denial behind me changed me for the better and initiated an amazing growth process. Being able to see and deal with my fears helped me help my father through the hardships that were to come.

It may take an incident, accident, a visit from the police, or trip to the ER before we can shrug our way out from under denial and take charge. In our case, I'm glad that nothing worse happened – that nobody was hurt or killed because of our inability to face the truth. Going against denial, however, meant going against a lifetime of training in the subtleties and fine points of disavowing reality.

It's important to at least be aware of our denial, even if we can't yet force ourselves to act. But eventually, we will be asked to lead the way by accepting the responsibility of addressing, managing, and being honest about the emotional and physical realities of the situation.

A Few Things I Figured Out.

- Denial is a natural, physiological response to shocks, events, and changes. It can help the mind and body adjust gradually to a difficult situation and, as such, is not a bad thing. When it becomes a way of life, however, and puts others at risk, it becomes dangerous. When a loved one becomes ill it can take an immense amount of physical and emotional energy just to see and name the walls hiding the truth before we can begin to break them down. It is essential for everyone's safety and well-being, however.

- Your family structure may be based on denial, and it may have served a purpose in the past. Be the one who begins to break the denial cycle. Now is the time to face as many of the relationship dynamics between you and your parent(s), spouse, and family members as possible: emotions, hierarchy, communication issues - all of it. It is time for open, honest discussion about what is happening, what will happen, and what can be done about it.

- Keep an eye out for poor grooming habits, especially if your loved one has always been proud of their physical appearance. Look for signs of poor nutrition or eating habits, changes in weight or dental health. If possible, go to their home and assess how they have been living and how their environment looks, feels, and smells to you. Look for confusion in speaking, repetition, answering questions strangely or an inability to answer simple questions at all.

Look for changes in attitude, confusion in doing simple tasks or an inability to do things they have done repeatedly for years. Be aware of sudden paranoia, and excuses for not going out or performing a task. Not all dementias include memory loss so keeping an eye out more for confusion, or aphasia (misuse of words), or repetition can be more useful. Inability or forgetting to pay bills, manage finances, or organize tasks can also be a sign.

- A situation may go downhill relatively quickly. Don't let the fact that they seemed fine a month before preclude believing there's a new, serious situation. People with dementia are highly skilled at concealing their symptoms.

- A short visit may not be long enough to show out-of-state family the extent of the dysfunction. If there are doubting family members, try to have them spend several days with the sufferer, to get a true idea of symptoms and problems. Try to speak with doctors independently of the care receiver to discuss symptoms and options for care and intervention. Above all, don't procrastinate if you feel something is wrong; be persistent in the face of denial or subterfuge.

3.

We Are Not in Kansas Anymore.

"Toto, I don't think we're in Kansas, anymore!" Dorothy, *The Wizard of Oz.*

So here you are. You've faced your denial and realized that something needs to be done – steps need to be taken. Congratulations. Your next problem is deciding what those steps need to be and, more importantly, how you are going to convince your loved one, and perhaps other family members, that things will no longer be how they used to be. The topography has changed. We are not in Kansas anymore but in some other country altogether where many things will change and roles will be exchanged. But how to do it? How to break through **their** denial?

Once my sister and I stopped denying reality, and began to work through both our horror at the situation and our complete lethargy around dealing with it, we realized we had no idea what to do. Because organizing physical and financial needs in the face of cognitive decline was a complete mystery to us, a friend referred us to a Geriatric Care Manager to help us make sense of what was happening and how we needed to respond to it. Geriatric Care Managers are generally nurses or health care specialists who are trained in geriatric issues and are usually licensed. They will assess the individual and determine their health and care needs, provide information and essential resources, assist in organizing medical, legal, and business affairs, and explain choices and options clearly.

We hired Kathryn Barrett, an eldercare advocate, registered nurse, and caremanager. She had made a career out of stepping into chaotic situations just like ours and making them run smoothly. She got to work right away, meeting with us and our father, gently and slowly determining his mental and physical state and attempting to get a sense of what his financial and legal status was. She had to work slowly because Dad was still in full denial about everything, including his mental state, our mental states, and the state of his affairs.

We told Dad that we had found a care-manager to help us deal with the situation and that we would be "helping" him in the future with his finances, self-care, and housing, something he reluctantly agreed with. The great thing about Kathryn was how very kind she was; she truly cared for Dad and his well-being, and she really included him in decisions and showed how much she respected him.

In a remarkably short time, Kathryn was able to sign our father up for Social Security and Medicare, something he had neglected to do even though he had turned sixty-five. She convinced him to let her bring in an accountant to go through his files and paperwork in order to attempt to get his affairs in order. Kathryn helped us create a care plan for Dad as well as a tentative schedule for what needed to be accomplished over several months – what was urgent, and what could wait.

I truly believe there is no way we would have succeeded without Kathryn. Since we conjectured that he must have some sort of cognitive failure, we hauled him to the doctor to determine the type, and to begin to address the physical and mental health issues that had resulted from solitary living, poor nutrition, and a mold-filled home. I was struggling with my own feelings about the situation - justifiably afraid of how it would most certainly impact my life.

I had a difficult enough time as it was managing my own life – trying to support myself while dealing with my chronic pain condition. I knew I could be facing hours and hours of energy and time addressing his needs that I wasn't sure I had to spare. I was also angry at Dad's continued efforts to make the process more difficult, in addition to the fact that he had allowed himself and his affairs to disintegrate so far.

It was so tough to yank him out of his denial so that together we could come to terms with what was happening and how to deal with it. He continued to believe staunchly that there was no disease, having spent so long covering up the cognitive and self-care difficulties he was experiencing that it could be like pulling teeth to get him to admit that there even was a problem, let alone discuss a solution that might need to be organized and then paid for.

In a manner very common to dementia sufferers, he would list things he was still capable of and insist on line-by-line descriptions of problems, which he would then refute one by one. My father had become a master at managing and masking his situation, and it was an uphill battle breaking through that mask.

When I received the second call from the police, informing me in the middle of the night that my father had been found disoriented and wandering yet again far from his home and had been conveyed to the emergency room in a Seattle hospital, she went immediately to the hospital to be with him. She found him shivering, disoriented, and upset.

Until that point, we had let him stay home alone, hoping that nothing serious would happen until we were further along in our plans. I believe it was at this moment that we all   realized that taking more aggressive action was absolutely essential. We were goaded along by the fact that the officer told me sternly that they had now opened a file on my father and his situation, that we were expected to deal with the problem, and that they would be watching to make sure it was handled and he was cared for.

*

Obviously, Dad could no longer live independently, subsisting on bread sandwiches and cookies, surrounded by hoarded newspapers and plastic. We had tentatively explored a few facilities, with the thought of moving Dad in as soon as possible, but none of them seemed appropriate yet for where he was physically and emotionally. What we really wanted was for him to remain in the familiar environment of his home. We surmised that being in his own house would probably make him and his illness easier to deal with, and might prolong whatever lucidity he could hold on to.

However, neither my sister nor I was willing or able, for various reasons, to move in with Dad and care for him, which meant we would need to find a twenty-four hour, in-home caregiver, something else we had absolutely no experience with. We told him that he absolutely had to have someone living with him – a conversation that did not go well. He again denied strenuously that there was anything wrong and protested that he didn't trust anyone to be in the house.

With Kathryn's help, we discussed our various options. We could find our own aide by advertising or other means, which meant employing and paying them privately, dealing with such things as insurance and governmental rules and regulations, and finding an alternate or filling in ourselves in the case of illness or inability to work. Or we could hire an agency to provide us with caregivers which meant all employment issues would be handled for us, and the agency would be responsible for providing alternate aides as necessary.

After much discussion, we decided on the latter and our care-manager referred us to an agency she had worked with before. She called them immediately and set up a meeting the next day with the agency director and an aide that the director thought might work. It was on that cold day in Dad's living room where we first met Del, an angel in the shape of a kind and jovial Filipino gentleman. Finding Del was a monumental stroke of good luck – one that I'm afraid doesn't happen to many families. I have since heard stories about hired caregivers practically becoming family members, they are so loved and trusted, but it is still rare. To say that, in many ways, Del became as close as a brother to dad, would not be an exaggeration.

Del was in his early sixties and spoke in a heavily-accented voice that was seldom above a raspy whisper due to some throat surgery he had undergone years earlier. It could be difficult at times to understand what he was saying, but it was never difficult to understand the compassion and friendliness he lavished on Dad.

Living in his own home gave my father the illusion of independence and allowed him to use the abilities and faculties that he still possessed. He and I both knew that it also allowed him to hold on to who and what he was for a little bit longer; the house kept him together, in a way, and he felt safe. Del was the person who addressed many of the health and safety issues affecting Dad. He cleaned out much of Dad's hoarded mess, sneaking it out of the house when my father was sleeping when necessary. He commenced filling Dad up with tasty, nutritious meals.

Del dealt with Dad's wandering by hanging bells on the front door of the house, alerting him to Dad's departure so that he could join him or redirect him to another activity. He also began taking Dad on walks that lasted for hours, an essential activity that tired Dad out and used up some of his nervous energy. Del ended up losing several pounds and getting into shape as a result of the walks. It was obvious that he really cared for Dad, and in turn, Dad began to care for and depend on Del, who became his constant touchstone in a world always changing due to disease.

Del was a god-send, and we thanked our lucky stars he had been the one chosen to help our father. He took Dad to church every Sunday and to his weekly adult day care, which consisted of a support group meeting, activities, and a lunch, and kept him company while he was there. Del took Dad to meet his own family so they could spend time with his grandchildren, which Dad enjoyed tremendously. They took long drives everywhere, just because Dad loved being in the car, and were always talking about some adventure they had just had – some park visited.

I think one of the reasons he succeeded with my suspicious, solitary, and depressed father was because he refused to be ignored or disliked. He was constantly patting Dad's shoulder or putting an arm around him, arm-wrestling or mock-fighting him, or poking and prodding him in some way to get him out of a bad mood and to get him talking. You couldn't ignore or hide from Del, and in the end I believe that Dad started to like him and interact with him out of pure self-defense.

I also believe that in many unobtrusive ways Del helped my father continue to feel like a person and a man by talking to him and treating him like a normal adult. The physical interactions, strength contests, and consulting with him about his wishes, all conspired to help Dad feel like he still existed in the world. He never overtly treated Dad like a diseased or demented person, and always dealt with him respectfully, and it is for this that I think I am most grateful to Del. That and the plain fact that Dad was safe with him, which reduced my stress and worry and gave me the space to begin addressing all of the financial and legal issues that still remained.

The simple fact that Dad now had someone living with him, something he would have been *horrified* by if he was in his right mind, was a huge sign, if I needed one, that we were no longer in Kansas. As a result of Dad's crisis, I had been forced to step in and start a fight I wanted no part of. I had always suspected that anything to do with taking over my father's life would be an exhausting, uphill battle – and here I was, only at the beginning.

*

It can be so difficult to know when and how much to intercede when faced with a loved one who appears to be suffering. We don't want to needlessly hurt them or make them feel attacked or marginalized, however we want them to be safe. It can be difficult to find a balance between pushing in too much, too soon, and hanging back too much. We fear disapproval or embarrassment, and are nervous about making a wrong decision. Perhaps our loved ones refuse to discuss certain topics or accept our assessment of the situation.

I tell people that the best rule of thumb when deciding how and when to assume more control is to try always to act in the care receiver's best interest. While it is perfectly normal to have your own ideas, needs, and priorities, don't confuse them with your loved ones'. You may have to move slowly at first and you may find that frustrating. There is a line between being overbearing and neglectful; navigate it carefully until it is evident that full interference is necessary. Remember that there is a difference between exchanging roles and authority with your parent and treating your parent like a child.

Your loved ones will be having their own difficult feelings about the situation and you will need to help them without imposing your feelings on theirs. Illness or old age is stealing who they are, including what they used to do and be for you and vice versa, and this is something to be grieved. It can be incredibly hard for a parent to accept dependence on their child, or a spouse on another spouse. It can be hard to admit to needing help and hard to accept it from someone else, especially if that someone was previously in a more dependent, inferior role.

We all fear loss of mental, bodily, and financial control, so hopefully we can understand and empathize with a loved ones' struggle to avoid it. There is a definite personal stigma against being a burden to your loved ones, to friends, or to society – a perception that can lead to isolation, stress, and waiting too long to speak out. Having to accept dependency after years of self-governance, productivity, and decision-making is a very difficult process.

It is just so important to stay patient and keep talking - keep trying to have the conversation with your loved one, even though they may not want to. At one point, we had to have a conversation with Kathryn about payment for her services since my dad refused to sign her contract or write her a check. She was willing to table the question of her contract for the few weeks it took us to convince (lovingly coerce) Dad into paying her. At other times, we just did as much as we could *around* Dad.

When it comes to the other people involved, like friends and family, it may be hard to understand why they try to remain so firmly in denial since you feel that you have finally accepted the situation. There may be those who will fight you on the diagnosis, which can complicate the situation and your life. They may refuse to believe it, either because the sufferer doesn't look or act sick, because they don't spend enough close time with the sufferer to see the symptoms, or simply because they don't want to face the changes that must take place within the family from a dementia diagnosis.

Siblings may not want to believe that there could be anything wrong with a parent. They may accuse you of worrying too much or having ulterior motives. They may fight you over money, time, responsibility, and even past events and emotional struggles. Siblings may also be reluctant to buck the family roles assigned to them, or may insist you stay in yours! Forums, books, and blogs are full of people talking about their loved ones refusal to accept the realities of their situation. They detail their fear and frustration that nothing seems to get through, that their family member won't accept help, won't accept suggestions about safer ways to live or handle money, won't listen to concerns.

*

The best thing you can do for yourself and your loved one is to have your own plan. It is not a matter of *if* the crisis will come but *when*. Expect the best and plan for the worst has become my motto. Gather as much information as possible about resources in your area, about decisions that you may be required to make, and what legal and financial options you may have. I can only wish I'd been so prepared. Look for facilities in your area that would work for the situation and your family. You're not agreeing to anything by just looking around. Investigate respite care and adult day programs that might work for your loved one. Investigate local Meals-on-Wheels programs, and in-home care services.

Like we did with our loved one, you may have to force your loved one to accept an in-home caregiver, or at least some part-time help, but be prepared for a struggle. Older people have a hard time giving up control of their homes, and may resent the intrusion of a home care aide. Unless you are prepared to move in with your loved one yourself, having the difficult conversation and telling them they must have help in order to keep them safe is necessary. Like us, you'll have to consider how you want to manage that care. Fortunately, there are many excellent in-home care agencies around to choose from. They can be expensive but the benefit is that *they* will be the one managing the workers – you have enough on your plate managing your loved one! If one aide can't come, they will arrange for another. All insurance, taxes, etc. are managed by the service.

If you decide to manage your own caregiver, which can be cheaper, be aware that you'll have to advertise for and interview that person and arrange for pay, taxes, schedule, etc. After that, be prepared for the possibility that a few different aides may need to be hired before one that suits your loved one is found. We were lucky with Del.

There is no right way to arrange for care, there's just the way that works best for you and your loved one. The important thing is to have a few options and a lot of information ready for the moment when your loved one and your family exit denial and enter the real world.

A Few Things I Figured Out.

- According to the Family Caregiving Alliance, the first steps for a new caregiver are as follows: start with a diagnosis; talk about health, housing, financial, and legal issues; invite family, friends, and your community into the situation; take advantage of community resources; find support for yourself; create a flexible care plan.

- Keep a private journal or notebook of behaviors that you see, symptoms that change, medications that are taken or not taken – the general progression of the disease. This can help when you are speaking to the doctor and your care receiver is assuring them that everything is fine when it obviously isn't! This can be an extremely valuable resource, as well as proof of what you are observing. You might also consider quietly videotaping symptoms and behaviors so that you have proof to show doctors.

- Don't be afraid to ask for help. Most of us don't have any experience in illness or caregiving. There are many people and agencies who specialize in what these choices are, how to know what you need, and how to go about finding it. Geriatric care managers, physicians and nurses, social workers, city or county agencies on aging and disability, and many good web sites are available and possess a lot of good information. Find out if there's anyone you know who has gone through something similar and ask for their advice and recommendations. Don't be afraid to be flexible and explore every housing and care option available to you. Something that might not have been appropriate before or which might not have occurred to you could be the choice you're looking for now.

- Caregiver support groups can be a great source of information, resources, medical options and how to find good doctors. Calling the facilitator of the group nearest you can be an invaluable way to get started on your information gathering. They may refer you to people in the group, who will also be a fantastic resource since they have been doing everything you are about to do! You can get great referrals for doctors and hospitals, advice on medications, and referrals for good facilities. Even if the group isn't close enough for you to attend, you may still get information that you need about resources in your relative area.

- Have your own plan and keep it secret as necessary. Even if you can't break your loved one out of denial at least you will be prepared with some options. Look up possible diagnoses, symptoms, plans of care, and medications. Investigate doctors local to you or your loved one that might be able to help. Investigate legal and financial issues and solutions. Look up potential living facilities, respite facilities, nursing facilities, adult day care, support organizations, meal delivery systems, organizations on aging and disease, in-home care businesses, and care managers in your respective areas. You won't be able to plan for everything, of course, but you will be in possession of your greatest asset and most powerful tool – information. Don't wait until you get a call from the police at three o'clock on a January morning, telling you that your loved one has just fallen and broken a hip and what do you plan to do about it?

- Don't hesitate to let an aide or caregiver go who you no longer trust or are able to work with. When hiring a stranger, perform the most thorough interview possible; create a checklist for your interview to assess the applicant and have questions prepared ahead of time; always ask for and check resumes and references. Above all, you must trust your instincts and gut feelings. You must decide what you can live with in terms of personal quirks, requirements, or habits of a private caregiver, i.e. insisting caregiver not be a smoker. Unless you are supernaturally lucky, you will probably face a few staff challenges. Always have a back-up plan -- or two -- in case of problems like illness or emergency. Remember that if you hire a caregiver privately, you will be responsible for finding a replacement for sick/vacation days.

4.

Family Caregiving is All Relative.

"A dysfunctional family is any family with more than one person in it."
Mary Karr

One of the biggest problems when my father started needing my help rested in the ways in which he had cared for <u>me</u> – or not cared for me, as the case may be. His perpetual depressive behavior, his workaholism and inability to relate to me, and his adherence to Christian Science were all things that had damaged me and made me reluctant to even have him in my life, let alone give him care. The issue I had the most problem with – which was standing in the way of my taking on his care - was connected to the Christian Science. Because of his adherence to his religion, he had abandoned me during a very real hour of need, when I was very ill.

My struggle with chronic illness began the summer between my Junior and Senior years in college. I was twenty-one and living at home, and I kept feeling incredibly tired and sick with a constant low-grade fever. As Christian Scientists we had not grown up in the medical system. I had no pediatrician to consult or any real idea of where to go to get help and so my illness progressed. Although I was living at home, my father was caught up in his own private world, seeming completely oblivious to what was happening to me. I remember once telling him I wasn't feeling well, but the rules against admitting illness were too strong for me to go into detail during our conversation and he did nothing.

There wasn't much pain at first, just a lot of discomfort and exhaustion. I had fevers and night sweats and a rash. I was having trouble eating and was losing a lot of weight. It was the fevers, constantly rising and breaking that really wore me out. Day and night the fever spiked and broke repeatedly so that I was either sweaty, cold, clammy, or burning up. I spent all day and every evening on the couch in the living room while Dad got up and went to work, came home, made himself dinner and puttered around the house.

After a few months, the pain started. My elbows completely froze up then my knees began to swell and stiffen until it was agony sitting down or getting up. It took me ages to get to the bathroom, nerve myself up to sit down on the toilet, and then nerve myself to get back up. My feet were in such pain I could hardly walk, and my knuckles were swollen. One pinky finger became permanently fused. The rest of my joints were constantly hot and stiff and I was eating Advil by the handful, because it was all I had to reduce the pain.

My friend finally took me to an Urgent Care Center. They gave me the business card of a local internist, and I made an appointment as quickly as I could. What followed were weeks of doctor's visits, blood draws, MRIs and other expensive tests, and emergency prescriptions of steroids. In the end, we narrowed it down to Rheumatoid arthritis, one of a class of autoimmune disorders that can cause severe joint inflammation and deformation, muscle, joint, and tissue pain, severe fatigue, fevers, rashes, and other not-so-charming symptoms.

Our immune systems are wonderful things, specifically designed to recognize, target, and eradicate viruses, bacteria, or other types of nasty invaders floating around amongst the cells of the body. An autoimmune disorder, so-called because the body's own immune system perceives a threat that may actually not exist and begins to attack its own cells and other systems, can cause serious illness and dysfunction. My autoimmune system is always activated, alert against an intruder that doesn't exist, striving to solidify my body and freeze my joints.

There are several variations of the disorder, including rheumatoid arthritis, lupus, ankylosing spondylitis, and, possibly, fibromyalgia. They all involve some level of organ damage, joint and tissue inflammation, pain, and fatigue, among other problems. Many people have identified a loved one's death, an accident, an illness, or other stressful event as an initiating factor to successive autoimmune problems. Sometimes, we just get unlucky.

Believe me when I say that it has not been an easy thing to live with. I wish now that I could have broken my family's rules about illness and spoken up for myself earlier, found a doctor, and gotten help because the damage, both emotional and physical, would last the rest of my life. When I told my dad my about my diagnosis and that I would be pursuing medical treatment, he essentially turned his back on me.

He said that only the Christian Science Church could do anything for me and he begged me to come back to the church with him. He was certain I would find no help with doctors or medication, and apparently, he wasn't even willing to help me or support me while I investigated the possibilities. There was nothing he could do for me. It was in that moment that I felt truly abandoned by my only remaining parent.

When my father's illness worsened, and it looked like I would need to be even more involved in his care than just paying his bills and finding someone to live with him, I faced a real quandary. How could I reconcile these facts of my childhood, along with my natural anger and resentment towards him, with the fact that he now needed my care?

*

With help, and time, I was able to come to terms with our shared past in order to start helping my dad. We found him 24-hour care, and I began dealing with everything else – bills, doctor visits, legal matters, etc. Six months or so after the initial panic and the denial and Del moving in, Dad's life was running more smoothly, however, there was still a lot of work to do, which I was doing while maintaining a full-time job. I took a hard look at the time and energy I was putting in dealing with Dad and his affairs, as well as the fact that Dad's disease was progressing. I was working and living about forty minutes away, but was spending in at least a day a week at Dad's house, struggling with financial issues or taking him to the doctor.

He had Del, of course, to help him, but I was still exhausting myself organizing his life and my own – something I couldn't afford to do with my chronic illness. The way I had my life organized needed to change and a daring solution occurred to me. I could quit my job and move in with Dad as his caregiver two days a week, ensuring I was on the spot to handle tasks and problem. I also wanted to keep a closer eye on Dad's health and changes in his disease and could do that better if I saw him regularly.

I went over the pros and cons endlessly – in my head, with my friends, with my sister, and with my therapist. The objections against caring for him were considerable, and legitimate. I would be giving up a job that I loved, and living two nights a week in the broken-down house that I hated. In many ways, it felt like I would be rewarding bad behavior – letting him get away with hurting me in the past, and letting him off the hook for leaving his life in an absolute mess. I would have to face up to the reality that he had not been the parent I wanted or needed, and that now he would never be that parent. I would never be able to get my needs met by him in an appropriate manner, and he would most likely never be able to acknowledge the ways that he had hurt me. We would never have the relationship we might have had.

My therapist helped me negotiate the ways in which I could accept these new changes. She reminded me that every time we discussed the possibilities, a common refrain of mine was always that I didn't want to miss anything about Dad's situation. I was constantly afraid I would miss some bit of connection, feeling, history or information that might emerge from Dad in his new state. I wanted to bear witness to as much of what was happening as possible, and I didn't want to look back later in regret that I hadn't been present. It seemed to both of us to be a very good reason to do what I was contemplating – being present in these last months and years of my father's lucidity.

I knew it might also give me a chance to participate in some sort of new relationship with him. There might be an opportunity to talk to him about the ways I felt he'd let me down or damaged me. It was possible I could get an apology or at least the feeling that I'd been heard. Perhaps we could share ourselves with each other in ways we'd never done before.

My therapist and I discussed the reality that there was no way I was taking the job unless there was some sort of exchange, not only for my valuable energy and time, but to redress the fact that I was essentially caring for a parent who had neglected to care for me. Being paid for my services was an essential part of the scheme so that I didn't feel I was giving everything away and getting nothing in return. The arrangement could also benefit me financially. I would essentially be working for Dad for forty-eight hours straight, since I would be sleeping there two nights, and it was possible he could pay me more than I was currently making to do it. I was unsure, however, whether I was ready to change my life so drastically.

Although his finances were still far from organized, we had finally determined that Dad had quite a bit of money, enough to pay me for my work. Since his money was so important to him – almost more important than his family - making him spend some of it also helped me feel some justice. Although I realize that unfortunately there aren't that many families with the kind of financial freedom we had, I tell caregivers that *some* sort of energy exchange is really important. If it can't be a salary, then maybe free rent or other assistance of some kind.

My therapist assured me she would be right there with me through the entire process, and I trusted her to help me. Together, we could hopefully get Dad the care he needed, while helping me work through the events and emotions of the past and begin the process of transmuting it into something more beneficial to me. It would be up to me to accept and work through all of the grief and resentment and. In the end, the rewards of dealing with these old feelings, assuming my father's care and potentially forging a new relationship with him, outweighed the risks and the rage. I decided I wanted to do it.

I took the plunge and arranged to work one day a week for my boss and committed to giving up two days and nights a week to be Dad's live in caregiver. I knew I would get angry and sad at times, which I needed to be honest about. I also wanted it to be clear that I wasn't making this sacrifice because I was a good daughter, caring for her loving Father. On the contrary, since my father and I had a difficult relationship, it was important for me to recognize and put out in the open my feelings about the whole situation, and not just sweep them under the rug or deny their existence. My father was not a great father – and I was caring for him anyway, which later made me think about other caregivers and *their* issues with family. This is an issue that in some way affects almost all of the caregivers I talk to. It makes me ponder – what is a caregiver to do if one's family hasn't been, or isn't much, of a family?

*

Whether posted on internet forums and discussion groups, written about in blogs or memoirs, or just discussed among the caregivers I've met, family problems related to caregiving get a lot of airtime. Almost all caregivers have issues with family. It is endemic in family caregiving, because, of course, there are a lot of people involved. Whether we are talking about siblings, parents, spouses, or extended relations – family members seem to let caregivers down more than anybody else.

Caregivers complain about siblings and other family members that refuse to help out, are absent or uncaring; step-children that are dismissive, in denial, or causing legal or care obstructions; or having to give care to spouses that were or are abusive, or to parents that refuse to accept help, cede control, or are abusive. In blog posts and forums they ask for advice about, cry about, and rant about these people, complaining about family members, usually siblings, who repeatedly let them, and an ill parent, down.

They describe people who are in denial about the reality of the illness, or who don't have a good relationship with the care receiver, or who choose to go their own way and do their own thing, or who simply don't seem to care. Caregivers also describe family members that crave complete control, who legally shut them out of decisions and knowledge. There is every combination of family dysfunction imaginable. Which begs the question: if we are constantly told that blood is thicker than water, and that we can always count on or turn to family, and that family is who has to take you in when you show up on the front door… why are there so many problems with "family caregiving?"

Let's be honest here. Despite the whole blood and water thing, from the dawn of time, family members have been lying to each other, betraying each other, abandoning each other, and even bashing each other's heads in – just ask Cain and Abel. Many of us have been abused, neglected, ignored, or betrayed by members of our family. The real, unspoken truth is that "family" can treat you, desert you, and take advantage of you worse than any friend, acquaintance, or colleague – which is a truth most people would like to forget or sweep under the carpet. It is just as likely that family members did not or do not, have close, loving bonds and did not or do not support or care for each other. And yet, "family" is still touted as the best thing since sliced bread.

As a society, we are taught to believe in the family unit, which is to say the idea that we can always rely on our family for love, support, and assistance. We want to think, and popular media supports, the myth that they will always be there for us when nobody else is and that all families band together and get along. This is not a bad thing to believe, exactly, but the problem is that given enough time and/or stress, the myth that is family inevitably starts to come apart at the seams, revealing huge gaps, frayed connections, and poor support.

This is a bottom line reality when a whole new paradigm of need and responsibility like caregiving hits a family – relying on the myth of family may not work. Sometimes family fails us, and it happens more often than the world realizes. I think it is so important to dispel the myth of family unity and unconditional love and support as much as possible when I speak to caregivers in order to normalize as much as possible their very real perceptions and experiences: experiences such as the difficulty of caring for an unloving parent, lack of involvement by siblings, family dissention and disparity of effort among family members, even problems like theft, betrayal, and legal battles.

I always ask caregivers whether they have any family who can help them because we think of family as the first line of assistance in a crisis situation, and I know that if they *have* family, they are going to need to be brought in to give their help. Some families are just small or are not in contact with each other, so I'm not surprised when a caregiver says they don't have family help. But other caregivers tell me they have large families – either several children, or several siblings, and sometimes even extended family close by. Regardless of this information, I am also not surprised to hear that the caregiver is struggling on alone or with one family member to help.

*

It's true that we all have roles to fill within our family network that allow the family to continue smoothly, and we fill those roles according to societal norms and established family scripts. We rely on the roles we fill for our sense of identity and we often invest in them heavily, and we rely on others to continue to fill their roles appropriately. We want family members to do and be what they've always done and been and we are more comfortable when everyone remains in the positions to which we've become accustomed.

Positions such as; parents must be independent and self-reliant, and take care of their children who are dependent on, or at least, subservient to, their parents. One sibling may be the peacemaker of the family, and tries to get everyone to get together and get along (this was me.) One member of the family can be the popular, outgoing one, another is the troublemaker. Maintaining our roles may help families function in normal, day to day life, but sometimes, situations or events that are outside our control change the entire structure of a family. Roles are ended, altered, or created based on the new circumstances, causing mental and emotional challenges.

A crisis like a family member needing care can bring out the best in people, helping to foster love, cooperation and courage. It can also cause some family members to become entrenched in old, negative patterns and roles and it can cause others to rise above themselves and the situation in transcendent ways. Some individuals will be able to face change, step outside of accepted behaviors, expectations, and obligations, and rearrange the family structure. Some individuals will not.

Crisis situations can put people on their best behavior and make them amenable to working together, but it is unrealistic to think behavior like this can hold for very long. Family belief and behavior patterns can run deep, and they do not just disappear because there is suddenly a serious situation to be dealt with. Inevitably, as the urgency of the situation fades, needs are managed, and a structure of care is established, problems set in and good behavior fades.

A situation involving long-term illness, caregiving, decision-making, and financial issues unavoidably requires frequent and often emotional communication around the subjects of family roles, compromise, difficult health and financial choices, and sacrifice. A family caregiving experience can damage and/or destroy a family. Different family members may act and react differently, express their own opinions and judgments, form alliances, regress into old roles and take stands, or abandon the situation altogether. Let's face it, we may have lived with these people for years but that doesn't mean we know, or understand, everything about them.

Old wounds and unresolved issues that have lain dormant for many years may surface under the pressure of new demands and a changed reality. This can rip off the bandage of civility and expose dysfunction, anger, and grief to the open air. The reality is that relationships are difficult and it is during these intense, challenging situations that the concept of family is tested, harshly strained, and pushed to breaking point.

*

Our society has changed so much since the early part of the century when family members stayed together, and marriages persisted. People live longer, marry multiple times, and may have multiple families, which can lead to more people to cause complications and dissent. Divorces, remarriages, and blended families means more people in the mix, along with their opinions, beliefs, reactions, and judgments.

Second wives fight to care for husbands in the face of the dislike and disapproval of step-children, or step-children help their mom care for a step-dad because his children are in denial. Men and women care for their ex-wives and ex-husbands because there is no one else willing or present. Adult children struggle against second spouses to act on behalf of or care for parents.

Women with multiple adult children may soldier on with a husband's care alone because the adult children are too busy to help, or just don't want to. Some family members will cause endless difficulties and throw up roadblocks to resolution, others may find untapped reserves of strength and courage. In some families everyone can pull together, split up responsibilities, and act, while in others one person is doing all the work while other siblings prevaricate, criticize or refuse to get involved at all.

I met one man who, while caring for his wife and helping her die, faced constant criticism and second-guessing from her extended family about her illness and his care choices. Her family had plenty to say about the whole situation but weren't willing to lend a hand; he was still left to do all the painful and boring work. And this happens a lot in families.

Some family members, not understanding the complexities of the situation, or just wanting to feel like they are involved, question every move, every decision, making things more difficult for the primary caregiver. Or family members put off participating in important decisions or actions; a choice which can cause financial or legal hardships. There are all sorts of ways that families can make things difficult. If you've ever tried to get a committee to work together, then you know how much harder it can be getting a family to do it.

Sibling relationships can become strained as family members negotiate new tasks and responsibilities; some family members may refuse to make further compromises or sacrifices, and others feel forced to sacrifice too much. One person, usually the closest in space or affection to the care receiver, may take charge and make decisions. Which can end in the situation I see so often on blog posts and forums, with one individual, who is not sure how it all happened, working alone and complaining about the actions – or lack thereof – of siblings.

Granted, there are "good" reasons why some family members are unable to be present. Some members may live too far away and are unable to assume responsibilities, while others may have family or work commitments, or even illnesses that make it difficult or impossible for them to help. There seem to be so many, however, who either just don't *know* how to care, or flat out don't want to. This can be both difficult and confusing, as if the demands of caregiving aren't enough.

*

And what about having to care for a parent who may not have been much of a parent? A friend and I were talking the other day about being caregivers. Six months ago, she invited her slightly ailing mother, with whom she has had a difficult relationship, to move in with her because her mother needed very nominal care but couldn't really live alone anymore. A few months later, what started out as mild ailments and transportation to doctor's appointments became full-blown issues.

My friend experienced her mother's infections and pneumonia, several hospital stays, an extended stay at a skilled nursing facility, and endured a sharp learning curve in medication, Medicare, Medicaid, and senior financial and legal issues. She was essentially thrown in to the deep end of caregiving, as so many of us are, and she was just starting to get her head above the water.

She has the type of job where she encounters, and talks to, lots of people and she mentioned how completely fed up she was getting with the comments she was receiving. The one that irritated her the most was the clichéd, and sometimes completely inaccurate, phrase, "Well, she cared for you, now it's your turn to care for her." I've heard this a lot, too, and I kind of hate it just as much as she does. The problem with the sentiment is that it's not always true – it is based on the myth of family togetherness.

Let's be real, some of us didn't have especially nurturing parents. In fact, a lot of us didn't and yet society doesn't really want us to talk about it. We both want to set these people straight by pointing out that our parents didn't, in fact, care for us, but caring for them is the right thing for us to do. I understand that people are trying to find a way to acknowledge that what we are doing is extraordinary, and difficult, and granted, it is probably not the time to inform them of our family history. However, these pat phrases can be more harmful than helpful.

I want to say to these people, "Who are you really talking about here? You? Because we seem to have stopped talking about me since this isn't MY history, and I'm not entirely sure it fits yours, either." Who are they trying to convince – them or us? I imagine these people might have their own slightly shady family history since very few people have had a perfect childhood with a perfect family. I suspect these sentiments are also generated out of deep fears that the same situation – having to care for a parent - may happen to them, and they will have to make the same uncomfortable choices we had to make. Sometimes, trying a scary situation on for size through somebody else, while whitewashing it at the same time, helps to make it a little less scary.

We usually don't talk about the fact that our parents may not have been good parents, but the reality remains – not all parents are successful at parenting. When we are children, we don't always realize exactly what is going on with our parents emotionally, nor what is missing from the care they provide us. Many of us have difficult relationships with our parents as adults because of things that happened, or didn't happen, in our childhoods; things that can range in severity from mild to completely abusive. It is a reality that most of us would probably say our parents had let us down, or hurt us, or didn't parent us in the way we needed.

There are so many reasons why parents are unable, or unwilling, to adequately care for their children, physically or emotionally, including; their own poor childhoods, religious beliefs, financial strictures, and mental or physical illness. The average parent is only human, they often do the best they can, but they are acting according to their own upbringings and belief systems, and are not always able to be the kind of parents we feel we really need.

There are also parents who, with great purpose and intent, attempt to damage and destroy their children. The scars from these types of upbringings can be formidable. I pity any adult child faced with a potential caregiving situation for a parent that was abusive because they are caught between what their parent needs and their own feelings of pain, grief, and anger. I firmly believe that there are more people in this situation than not – facing the emotional challenges of difficult family relationships while having to also give care. It's a fact that the ways in which we were parented or the actions of related adults in our lives in the past will affect our choices and feelings about caregiving.

There are many who have had it much worse than I; people who are facing the choice of caring for abusive parents, or parents who abandoned them. It is vital to acknowledge the absolute truth that who our parents were and how we were parented in the past affects us in the present - emotionally, mentally, and physically – regardless of whether there is a caregiving situation or not.

What if your parent *was* abusive? Neglectful? Uninterested? Conflicted about parenting? Absent? If you had a poor (or no) relationship with the person who now needs your care, you might have a difficult decision about whether you want to help. If you do help, you will definitely have feelings about it that you will need to be aware of. Essentially, you have two basic choices; either become their caregiver, or don't. There are variations and compromises but in the end, this really is what it boils down to.

All too often, it is assumed by outsiders that when there is a parental caregiving need, adult children will be able and willing to step in because of that bond. The unspoken reality is that there might not be a bond, or that adult child may decide they don't want to give care. This might or might not be a relatively easy choice for those who had steady, supportive, present parents. However, if you have not had the perfect childhood, the perfect parents, how are you supposed to feel when you are called upon to meet their needs, and what will you do?

Bringing oneself to give care to a parent who didn't provide it or who was actively abusive or neglectful is a difficult personal choice and can be a long-term, challenging issue. Why should you feel obligated to care for someone who mistreated you? I believe you should at least understand you have a choice. If you decide you just can't take care of parents who didn't care for you, I think that's your right. I believe it is okay to choose *not* to be there for someone who wasn't there for you.

People may judge you for your choice - you may even judge yourself - but the bottom line is that it is your choice that matters, and the world needs to respect it. Nobody can know what your childhood experience was or why you are making the choices you are making. You can't make this kind of choice capriciously or without counsel, and you shouldn't have to make it under the judgments or opinions of anyone but a close and trusted friend or family member.

If you decide that you *want* to give care, I recommend that you make the choice fully – it is essential that you be honest with yourself and your feelings, and about what you might want to get out of the situation. I also recommend that you find a good therapist or spiritual guide because there will be a lot of past and present issues and emotions that will come up during your caregiving tour of duty, and you should have help to deal with them. Anger, resentment, and fear are only a few of the things I can almost guarantee will come up

– dealing with them as they happen instead of stuffing them down is essential.

You must grieve that aging and disease are stealthily stealing away any possibility that they could have been different parents and could have been what you needed. With help you may be able to let go of who your parents were and who you may have wanted them to be and accept that they will never be able to go back and do things differently, which will be hard. (I recommend this to everyone, actually, not just caregivers!)

In addition, while you are grieving the parent they were and the chances that have been lost, you may also be grieving the fact that you are losing them as they are now. Regardless of how good or bad they were as a parent, they are still your parent - the person that holds your history and has been with you from the beginning. You must allow yourself to feel all of these conflicting feelings and work through them, instead of repressing or denying them.

*

This is not to say that it is *impossible* to navigate a caregiving situation with family, only that it is inherently difficult. The more open and honest the lines of communication and the more clear the expectations and responsibilities, the better. Encourage family members to be realistic about their agendas, abilities, and willingness to be involved. If you can't get them to do that, try to be realistic on their behalf, and set your tasks accordingly. Sometimes, families respond well to group meetings with a referee like a pastor, lawyer, doctor, or trusted family friend. Writing out what needs to be done and who might be willing to assume what task can be helpful.

Sometimes it can be a matter of finding out what people are good at and what they are willing to do and having them do it. If one family member lives far away but is good with money, for instance, have them balance the check book and pay bills. If a sibling can't face spending time with a care receiver, have that person do the laundry of grocery-shopping. Above all, and I want you to engrave this in your heart, you will never be able to change any member of your family. At all. Ever. Be honest with yourself.

Decide what you will put up with from your family, set clear boundaries if possible, and remember yourself, and your care receiver. You are doing this for good reasons of your own. We must be willing to carry on with our choice to be caregivers, regardless of the involvement of anyone else, knowing that every family member has their reasons for their actions, and they will get back what they put in. Hopefully, we are reaping the rewards of our caregiving, even though they may be few and far between.

Decide whether you want to care for the parent who was abusive or dismissive or wasn't present in your life. Make a choice about whether you want to care for a spouse who did not care for you. If there is no choice *but* you – no other family member who can do the job – decide what your boundaries are going to be. Require that you get paid or receive some other type of compensation. Most important of all, get support – someone to talk to – so that all the feelings don't get buried inside. It will never be simple, but you can make it work for you.

I'm not going to say that living with Dad and caring for him was easy going. From the start, I had many set-backs. It was difficult work and my emotional equilibrium has been rocked over and over. What I found, however, was that the honesty and the acceptance was making space for something new to happen between us. I was able to be brave and step past the roles we had always played for each other, and he was able, largely due to the effects of the disease, to be more open and loving than he ever had been. In effect, we created a whole new relationship between us; a relationship that was more about the present than the past.

Unfortunately, Dad's situation caused a rift between my sister and I, which I talk about in another chapter. Our relationship was not able to survive the expectations and realities of caring for my father. She chose not to be very involved and I felt the same bitterness and anger towards her lack of commitment that many others do. It has taken me many years to come to terms with her behavior and with what our relationship has become.

I think that as caregivers we can only do what we can do, according to our own lights and whatever moral and emotional compass we might have. In truth, we all choose to care for a family member for different reasons – there are as many caregiver stories as there are stars in the sky. I think that what is common to all caregivers, however, is our ability to somehow find the courage to choose to do what seems right to *us* – and then to do it.

It is unrealistic to believe that the experience that is family caregiving will ever be free of the dynamics and entanglements of the family. It is keeping the issue a secret, however, that is the problem. We want to know that we are not alone in our untenable situation, we want to feel that *our* family is not the only one that has failed, or is dysfunctional, or unable to put personal issues aside to pitch in and stand together through thick or thin like the myth says.

The myth of family is no longer acceptable. It can be emotionally destructive, demoralizing, and damaging because it leaves little room for honesty, fosters harmful expectations both of one's self and between family members, and can lead to physical and emotional consequences. Just knowing that other caregivers are experiencing the same problems with their families may be helpful to new caregivers who are struggling for some sense of the "normal." No two family experiences will ever be the same, nor will any two caregivers. Sometimes it makes me sad that there are enough caregivers with difficult family situations to need a chapter like this. My goal is only to break the myth that families are perfect and all-supportive and ever-present.

Maintaining a lack of honesty about family issues and relationships can be hurtful and unproductive just in normal life. Caregivers need to know the truth about what might happen so that they don't need to face the demands of caregiving while struggling with the disparity between their reality and what society would prefer to believe. Whether the reality of the situation is uncommunicative and uninvolved siblings; critical extended family members; or a complete breakdown of the family unit – we must be honest about it because it affects the health and wellbeing of the caregiver. If we can really look honestly at how the demands and emotions inherent in caregiving affect the family, then perhaps we can take steps to address it. We could separate the difficulties and challenges of having to give care to a loved one from the difficulties and challenges of family relationships and reduce the stress and frustration quotient by half. Just an idea.

A Few Things I Figured Out.

- Being in a family doesn't mean you have a close relationship with family members. My family didn't have strong relationships with each other and had no real communication structure – all of which really hindered the process of caring for my father. A caregiving situation can expose every single weak spot, fault line, and difficult dynamic that a family possesses. Family members just aren't always there for each other, and families don't always band together during a crisis. Acknowledging that this is what is actually 'normal' is the first step in being honest about family and caregiving. Breaking free of expectations and roles and relegating them to the past will help facilitate the caregiving process.

- Family dynamics can be frustrating and time-wasting and can render one ineffective and impotent. The first struggle to break through family issues in order to begin to have a useful discussion can be incredibly difficult but it may make it easier for everyone. Try to have meetings or discussions with as many family members as possible. If you are aware of the possibility of problems, ask a neutral third party to be present at the meeting: an extended family member, trusted friend, therapist, pastor, geriatric care manager, social worker, or lawyer. Sometimes it is necessary to have a witness who can see and hear things clearly without the emotional family complications. Make sure someone is taking notes and that the notes – and any plans - are read and agreed to by everyone.

- Did you, too, have a poor parent; a less than supportive family? Welcome to the club! Don't be fooled by Hallmark, there are more people like you than not, they just tend to keep quiet about it. Luckily, there are now more books out there, including memoirs about alcoholic, neglectful, or just poor parents, and about the difficulties of choosing to care, as well as ways to help you adjust. There are also many blogs, forums, and other on-line resources where people discuss these issues.

- It is each individual's choice whether or not to give care. No matter what you hear or what other people think, it is not as natural as, "They took care of you, now you take care of them." You have to choose what will be right for you. There may be judgment, from others as well as yourself, but whatever choice you make is valid and should be respected. Remember, there is no "right thing", only the right thing for you! Find yourself a good therapist, minister, or someone trusted to talk to. These are big, complex feelings and you are going to need help getting through them. Grief, anger, resentment, uncertainty, fear, and abandonment are just a few. Having to give care is big enough without dealing on your own with all the attendant emotions.

- Remember that others' coping methods differ and may conflict with yours. Sometimes it can simply be a matter of learning your family members' strengths and weaknesses and then using them in the right way at the appropriate time and situation; that way, everyone's needs have been met, everybody feels they have been useful or have been heard. A family member may really want to help but not know how. Be clear and upfront about possible needs and duties.

- As the primary caregiver, you may make decisions that are unpopular with the family. Others may have their own ideas of appropriate care; they might be influenced by old grudges and patterns, or they may simply be reacting out of guilt that they are not able, or do not want, to be caregiving. Be patient, try to listen, but be firm. You are the primary caregiver, you are the most involved and are likely most aware of the best interests of your loved one.

5.

Dementia - The Undiscovered Country.

"Everyone who is born holds dual citizenship, in the kingdom of the well and in the kingdom of the sick. Although we all prefer to use only the good passport, sooner or later each of us is obliged, at least for a spell, to identify ourselves as citizens of that other place." Susan Sontag

When I first became ill with my *own* illness, I wish that there had been someone there to explain what was going to happen, what was going to change, and how I might best survive. I wished this even more when Dad became ill, because I had so little experience with the uncharted territory that is dementia. I wish there had been someone there to welcome me to this new country; this country of illness and physical and mental dysfunction, where there is no normal. Where the rules are different from those I was once accustomed to and are ever-changing. Where the language shifts almost daily and can be confusing and incomprehensible, and the topography never remains the same.

I wish someone had told me that no matter who my dad and I used to be, or how familiar or comfortable we were in our old lives with our old desires and pastimes, or how well I knew him or the place he occupied in my life – that we would have to come to terms with the fact that everything had now altered and would only continue to do so. One is forever changed even by a short stay in the country of illness. Dad and I had our citizenship status irrevocably altered before we even realized it.

*

Living with Dad in this new land was an interesting experience. Every Sunday afternoon, I would pack a bag, leave my studio apartment and my two cats, and drive over to his (mildew-filled) house. I would greet Dad and Del, put my stuff in my room, and then have a quick chat with Del about what he and Dad had been up to, what groceries needed to be bought, and how he seemed to be feeling.

Del and I kept a spiral notebook in the kitchen of the house where we wrote down everything Dad had done and eaten and any change in symptoms, attitude, or behavior that we saw. We could also note if he seemed like he was getting sick or didn't like a particular meal or had refused his medication. This was helpful when we took him to the doctor and had to describe the progression of the disease. But we always kept in touch verbally, as well.

"Has he eaten?" "Oh yeah, we had chicken and potatoes for dinner. He enjoyed it." Del would say, then leave until Tuesday night. Dad and I would spend a little time together then he would wander down to his room and shut his door for the night.

The next morning, I would get up and have my breakfast and when I heard him stirring at about nine-thirty, I would start making his eggs or waffles or whatever I thought he'd like. After breakfast, it was time to run errands, go grocery shopping, go for a walk, or do whatever else I could think of to entertain him.

We spent a lot of time at our local tourist attractions and museums, including Boeing's Museum of Flight, a big favorite. We also walked almost every day, went out for lunch, or to the mall to watch people. I even took him bike riding and roller-blading a couple of times, which he was actually pretty good at.

After getting home from our outing each day, I left him in the living room with the newspaper, or to walk down to the lake shore, and I spent a few hours in my room, resting. I would make him dinner, we would have a nice evening eating and talking, and then he was off to bed early again. Late on Tuesday evening, Del would come back, we would again exchange a Dad update, and I was off – free for another five days. It was an existence unlike anything I had experienced before – like being a Gypsy.

I had been on my own since I graduated college, and being back in the family house two days a week, looking after Dad then moving back to my own apartment, was strange at best. At times, it was incredibly tedious and boring, at others, it was delightful and interesting. Most of the time, however, I felt the rightness of what I was doing – being with him in this new country, helping him go through this transformative experience – and, in a strange way, healing our relationship. Perhaps it couldn't have happened any other way.

Living with Dad, I had a front row seat to the changes dementia was making in him, and it was definitely a little difficult to watch him daily lose himself to something he couldn't even bring himself to name. It was hard for me to observe this incredibly smart, competent, and talented professional man whose entire being was slipping away from him, especially since he had fought so hard all of his life to control everything he could.

He valued and depended on control at all times. From his family to his feelings to his physicality, he strove to keep it all in check, subject to his will. Containment of emotions through self-discipline, mastery of the body through will and self-denial, and authority over his affairs through secrecy and self-sufficiency was everything for him. For him to lose control must have been terrifying.

He was in denial for the earlier, "lucid", stages of his illness and could not come to terms with the changes that were happening to him, which meant he was unwilling and unable to accept any comfort I might have given him around the horror of his situation. It broke my heart to have him walk up to me in the kitchen and ask why he could remember complex mathematical equations but got lost going from his bedroom to the living room. I could only reply that it was a consequence of his illness, although I knew he would immediately block out even the suggestion that he was ill.

Christian Scientists depend on the written word for healing and comfort, words they read to themselves, memorize, and internalize. Repeating Bible verses, hymns, prayers, and other texts in an effort to erase the erroneous belief in an illness or injury – negating what they don't want to believe in. I watched as the words he needed to proclaim his wellness and perfection were lost to him as he gradually lost the ability to read and comprehend the comforting texts.

He tried for a long time to force the ability to read and pray to come back, holding his Bible and other books, pretending he could still understand, undoubtedly repeating in his mind whatever fragments he remembered. His one concession to the *possibility* of a very slight problem with his memory was the constant possession of a little notebook and a pen wherever he went – usually tucked into the breast pocket of his shirt. I watched as he periodically filled up these little notebooks with abbreviated descriptions of his daily activities in his cramped, precise, engineer-trained printing. Details about meals eaten, places visited, things seen, the weather, and the people (myself or Del) who accompanied him as well as the cars they drove.

He always seemed slightly ashamed of this process, shielding the notebook from my eyes or writing when he was alone. He kept the filled notebooks in his dresser drawer, rubber-banded together. He also wrote accounts of each day's activities on his calendar under the appropriate date in an effort to document the days and events that were vanishing from his memory.

Sometimes I would sneak a look at these notebooks to see what he remembered or what he thought about the progress of his days. It was like reading a code. He was very interested in the food he was given and how it had tasted, sometimes writing down ingredients or the prices if it was in a restaurant. At times he seemed confused about who he had been with, mixing me up with another aide or noting that he had been with someone but couldn't remember who. It was a little hard to read that he didn't always know me.

It was also hard to see the truth, which was that he was forgetting so much and was so desperate to hold on to what he could. I've kept these notebooks in an effort to keep who he was during that time and as a way of understanding what he was thinking and feeling about his life. It must have been agonizing for him to dwell in this new place – to give up autonomy and independence and to have to be cared for like a child. To be monitored and told what to do and to watch others have to step in and help him. And, the absolute worst, to experience his mind no longer responding to his will and his wishes, and his body changing in ways he couldn't understand or accept.

*

Illnesses differ in magnitude, gravity of symptoms, and severity. They can, and do, affect the body, the mind, and the spirit, mutating all of these into unrecognizable shapes, and removing vital abilities and functions - sometimes temporarily, sometimes permanently. In fact, all illnesses reduce and remove something – even temporarily - whether it's the ability to move intentionally, to think clearly, to breathe deeply, or to live freely without assistance, fear, or hindrance. This has not changed since we began, as humans, to get ill. It is a gradual withdrawal from territory, an abnegation of autonomy, and sometimes feels like a forced loss of elements of humanity. To be ill is often to be in fear – it can mean loss, and rage, and despair.

Dementia, in particular, strikes at the heart of what we consider makes us an individual - makes us who we are. We think of it as just a memory stealer, which it is, but eventually it will steal everything else. Dementia brings with it fear: fear of the loss of love, the loss of the self, of purpose and of value. It changes so much about the sufferer. It will change who they are, how they think and feel, and how they behave – rewriting and deleting programs, reshuffling abilities, and permanently shutting down parts of the brain. Someday, your loved one will cease being the person you know, and they will cease to know themselves.

Dementia is essentially an umbrella term, meaning a lack of – or serious decrease in – two or more cognitive abilities. Cognitive abilities are mental functions that humans use to perceive, think, remember, communicate, and control our impulses. Dementia syndromes encompass a broad number of symptoms, including: loss of memory, mood changes, behavior changes, and problems with communication and reasoning.

Dementia surrenders are usually marked by physical and cognitive declines, which caregivers wait for in dread and resignation. A decline can be signified by the inability to remember details or events, a lack of self-care, difficulty walking or talking, dependency, and, devastatingly, lack of recognition of loved ones. At times these small hints of disintegration slide by unnoticed until a caregiver realizes something vital has altered. At other times, they are large and dramatic – impossible to ignore.

Dementia sufferers may also experience problems with attention and alertness, often have spatial disorientation and experience difficulty with "executive functions", cognitive processes that include working memory, reasoning, planning, and problem solving. This can include difficulty in planning ahead and coordinating mental activities.

These are all changes that dementia sufferers have no choice but to accept – and caregivers to watch. As caregivers, we can see how difficult it is as we go through these losses with our loved ones

– to *see* the changes and feel the effects of their gradual withdrawal from us. But imagine what it is like as a sufferer – to feel yourself slipping away little by little and know you weren't ever coming back. Remember that this person is losing their identity and, at least at first, is painfully aware of it. All that they are, feel, and know is slowly slipping away to be replaced with emptiness and humiliation, loss of value and loss of worth.

*

Suffice it to say that a caregiver for dementia will see anything and everything from their care receiver so it is best to be as prepared as possible. To help them, it is important to provide yourself with some sort of map. Start researching and exploring the symptoms and issues. Get as many facts and as much info about dementia as possible.

Dementia rarely takes place in a linear, logical disease progression. The symptoms and behaviors of dementia can and will vary. You may see forgetfulness, poor decision making, poor self-care, repetitive behaviors, paranoia and other delusions, elaborate hallucinations and illusions, aggression and shouting, wandering, eating off other people's plates, wandering into strange houses and businesses, inviting strangers into the home, and urinating and removing clothes in public.

Straitlaced fathers swearing and yelling; gentle mothers saying mean things and refusing to eat or get dressed; husbands threatening wives, sure that they are cheating on them or stealing from them; wives having elaborate hallucinations, talking to people that aren't there and seeing animals around the house. If I am asked whether this is "normal" for the disease, I can only say yes, that this is their new "normal", as much as I don't believe in that word. This is all part and parcel of dementia.

Some people experience dementia with more behavioral issues than others. Severe visual and non-visual hallucinations – seeing, hearing, or feeling something that isn't there – and illusions, a real object or person that the sufferer sees and interprets incorrectly. This can include dreaming and believing the dreams to be true. The sufferer may then interact with these phenomena, sometimes benignly, sometimes dangerously, often resulting in unsafe behaviors for the sufferer and the caregiver.

Dad came to me one morning, excited and somewhat distressed, with an elaborate story about a sailing trip he had just taken (although he no longer had a sailboat.) Apparently, he had been out in the boat by himself when a terrible storm blew up suddenly. Although he had fought against the wind and waves, the boat had eventually capsized and he had been lucky to get away from the wreck with his life! He couldn't believe it had happened, and neither could I, of course, as we stood together in the kitchen. I saw no need to shock or distress him by insisting it hadn't happened, and merely told him how sorry I was that such a thing had happened and how glad I was that he was safe.

This wasn't the only time that he saw things or had hallucinatory dreams. He called me late one night, anxious and agitated, and told me a convoluted tale about his caregiver insulting him, laughing at him, and even blowing smoke in his face and threatening him. My poor Father had barricaded himself into his room in fear. When I got there, the aide, a quiet and unassuming young man, was visibly upset and apologetic – it was obvious that nothing like what my father described had happened. I calmed him and sent him home, then went to check on Dad. I was finally able to soothe him and put him back to bed. I suspect he had been sleeping and had a vivid dream/illusion, woken up and been convinced that it was real.

For the most part, Dad was so quiet about what he was experiencing internally and in his mind that he could have been seeing things all the time and all over the place without me knowing about it. In fact he probably was seeing things all the time, it was only occasionally that information about it would slip out. I don't know if this was because of his denial of his illness and fear that if he said anything, it would lend credence to my assertions that he had dementia. It may also have been because he *knew* they might not actually be there and he didn't want to sound crazy.

Delusions – believing false perceptions to be true – can cause paranoia, suspicion, sadness, and anger. I have heard of sufferers accusing their caregivers of lying to them, stealing from them, being unfaithful, and abandoning them. These delusions can be persistent and disruptive, and can sometimes lead to combativeness, verbal abuse, and other acting-out behaviors. Dad was paranoid, but not aggressively so, and I didn't notice any other delusional behaviors, fortunately.

Aggression, both verbal and physical, fear, dark illusions and general acting-out can be common. Unfortunately, it appears that those who suffer from dementia trend towards darker memories, thoughts, and illusions so reactions can be negative. Some experts believe that this is a result of our primitive brain being hard-wired to remember things that can hurt us so we know to avoid them

As the disease progresses, behaviors and symptoms will change. Some behaviors may disappear while new ones take their place. Modesty often breaks down, leading to challenging behaviors involving sex and bodily functions. My ultra-modest, reserved Father began urinating in strange places such as potted plants and the corners of his room - something that, I'm sure, would have horrified him if he'd been aware. There are cases of dementia sufferers being arrested by police for what appeared to be public drunkenness. Recently a man was even shot and killed by police for waving what they thought was a weapon, which turned out to be a shoe.

The public can sometimes be uncomfortable with dementia's effects and manifestations, which can lead to denial and a lack of patience and empathy when faced with it in one's family or in public. It never really bothered me when I took Dad out and he acted a little oddly. I would usually order for him in restaurants, after helping him decide what he wanted. I always tried to engage him in the ordering process and waiters seemed to take it in stride.

At times he looked a little strange, having dressed himself, and there were times he didn't shower for a few days, but I chose not to make a big deal about it and allow him to maintain some dignity. I figured if it bothered someone else, it was their problem, not his and for the most part, people were understanding if he looked odd or smelled odd, made rude or questionable comments out loud, or repeated himself.

There were a few incidents where I had to pull someone aside to explain that he had dementia. A lot of websites now have cards that caregivers can download and hand out to members of the public explaining why their loved one is acting oddly, without the discomfort of having to explain the issue to people right in front of the sufferer. Most people are still unused to interacting with someone with dementia and are unprepared for its physical and emotional realities - even though it is becoming much more common and prevalent in awareness campaigns around Alzheimer's, and advertising for Assisted Living facilities with so-called Memory wings. There can still be a lack of understanding of the disease process, what the sufferer is feeling and experiencing, and why they are behaving as they are – even from those who have experience with it.

*

It is hard to know exactly how input and environments are affecting those with dementia, or how much they are absorbing. Environment seems to play a really significant role in the behavior and well-being of a dementia sufferer. Things like too much light or noise, too much bustle or stimulation, too many family members around, can be overwhelming for a dementia sufferer. Some care receivers enjoy watching a lot of television, finding the noise and pictures comforting. Some find the television agitating or over-stimulating, or the pictures may spark unpleasant memories. Watching the news or violent and fast-paced shows can make a care receiver anxious or even angry and can make it hard for them to sleep.

I was very careful about what I introduced into Dad's environment. We didn't have a television in the house, so he didn't watch that, and I played his favorite classical music when I could. Certain songs that came on the car radio would upset him so I kept it off, and I was careful what subjects I talked about. I rarely mentioned my mother, for example, because that seemed to agitate him a little. Eventually, his day care program became over-whelming for him because there were too many people – caregivers and care receivers. He could no longer cope. I also kept his room the way he liked it, with curtains drawn, so that the room was dark and cozy. Environment is not always going to be a factor in your care of a dementia sufferer, but for the most part, keeping the atmosphere less stimulating is a good practice.

In the last few years, I've watched Dad when people were talking to him and wondered what he was actually experiencing. There is an old cartoon that features a dog looking expectantly at her master, who is trying to talk to her or direct her to do something. From the point of view of the man, the dog is apparently listening intently, prepared to do exactly what he is asking, but from the dog's point of view, most of the man's words are incomprehensible, interspersed with the few words the dog actually understands like her name or "food" or "bad girl". The man is speaking English, but all the dog hears is meaningless noise.

I have wondered if, as his illness progressed, it became the same for Dad – random noises interspersed with recognizable words. Does he experience our conversation as coming to him through a tunnel, muffled or distant? Or are voices like a cloud of bees, swarming around him, noise meaning nothing. Is it annoying to listen to noise he doesn't understand, or peaceful, or just noise? I will never know except to hypothesize that reality as we know it just doesn't apply to those with dementia – the parameters just aren't the same in any way.

Another symptom that dementia sufferers can experience is called, "sundowning." This phenomena happens most often in the late afternoon, which leads some physicians to believe it might be related to one's circadian rhythm and changes in light. Dementia sufferers can become agitated, sad or more confused than normal, and they may act out more violently and more physically. This can be a difficult time for those with dementia, especially if caregivers or staff aren't aware of what's happening and treat the person's behavior as a problem. There are ways that sundowning behavior can be addressed without medication or increasing the agitation.

*

In the end, as I have said, life with dementia is all about relinquishing control. Care giver and care receiver will both have to surrender again and again and again as the situation evolves. If the body is a container for the soul - personality, experiences, beliefs, memories, loves - in short - everything an individual feels themselves to be - then dementia is the fissure in that container, allowing its precious contents to slowly leak out. Dementia removes memories and abilities, intelligence and awareness, confidence and the experience of emotions, and many of the other things that we consider make us human.

However, it might not be all bad. It can both rob you of moments, and give them to you like gifts. It can be simultaneously the worst and the best thing you have ever experienced together. A caregiver can perform a most sacred and important function when they collect and keep as much as possible of who and what their loved one was.

A dementia sufferer needs someone to hold who they are and remember their life. If you become a care-giver for someone, you can choose to become the living repository of much of what that person was or did, like an external hard drive saves and stores data. I became just such a repository - a memory holder and storehouse of as much as possible of what Dad was and is. I believe that tiny elements of what makes my dad who he is will remain within him until the very end, and I'll do my best to hold on to who he was, as well.

Long after he is gone, I will remember these facts and feelings so that he lives on in my memory. It is a gift to your loved one to listen to their stories, and to hold on to a little bit of their souls. My dad and I have certainly had our issues, but it comforts me to run these memories through my mind and tell the stories to my husband, because in that way, a little bit of Dad remains in other people, as well.

One of the stories Dad told most often in the early stages of his illness was about his work as a Boeing engineer. At one point, he was testing flight systems that he had helped design. He and a few colleagues would go up in the new plane and the pilot would go through various maneuvers to test whatever part of the plane they were working on.

There was one particular flight he seemed to remember more than any other, and he told me those details over and over: what the pilot did and said; the feeling of the plane in flight; the delight in fixing something that had been incorrect. Clearly, this period of his life was important to him, representing as it did the height of his intellectual and professional life. He would repeat the story over and over, with the same sense of delight and pride, and I tried to listen each time as if it was the first.

Things like this are all part of what makes up an individual who is slowly losing his individuality. The disease forced him to give up so much, and will eventually force him to give up everything. I can't control or change that for him, but I can hold on to some of what he was. I wanted to nurture and support the rich, well-established truth of his actual past experiences, achievements and loves, which were stored before the dementia.

Mostly, I tried at all times to let him be who he was – I wanted him to feel like an individual who mattered for as long as possible – that he had things to say that I wanted to hear. I wanted him to always feel as if I was on his side. It was the best way I could show him empathy and care for who he was now, not what he had been. It was part of how I saw, supported, and held on to, the Divine in my father. Being a caregiver for my father changed my life in ways I couldn't have imagined when I started. I was asked to come up higher, to have the courage to work through issues like anger and resentment, and to allow my Self to expand. It's been challenging and difficult and absolutely maddening – and at the very same time, it's been funny, deepening, and enlightening.

The whole process has been messy, angry, sad, annoying, irritating, lovely, and heartfelt. It was difficult to give up control, and find the humor in each situation, and it was hard to feel as if it was anything but a lot of hard work. However, I truly don't think I would be the person I am today if my father had not become ill and required my help. Caring for him helped me heal many things.

*

Coming into caregiving and the realities that go along with illness and dementia with prior expectations and assumptions only leads to disillusionment and disappointment. There are no definitive or failsafe ways to approach the emotional realities and complexities of the disease of dementia or the exigencies of giving care; there are no normal ways to handle the situations that will arise, the demands that will need to filled, and debilitating feelings that will manifest.

Caregivers and their receivers can learn together to be flexible and aware of what can, and will, occur so that they can navigate a way through each individual emotional of physical situation according to their abilities, needs, and environment. It is important to learn as much as possible about its progression, the symptoms and behaviors one can expect, and strategies that can help with care. Caregivers must be as educated and aware as possible about why something is happening, and what might be coming next.

The most important thing to remember, as caregivers are looking over their "maps to dementia" is that there are no "established" or "normal" dementia behaviors because, of course, this is not a "normal" disease. Be proactive in your expectations, which may limit surprise and unpreparedness when something new pops up. It is also incumbent on caregivers to advocate for our loved ones and continue to try to educate others on the realities of these diseases to alleviate fear and anxiety and promote understanding.

My heart goes out to all of the caregivers and care-takers experiencing routine, daily struggles with incredibly challenging dementia symptoms and behaviors. This place called illness is a baffling, difficult, and peculiar place to be; a place nobody would choose voluntarily. Caregiver and care receiver must learn together how to navigate it. It can be a challenge to accompany a loved one into their new country. All disease can be confusing, exhausting, and disheartening, for caregiver and care-taker alike, so be gentle with yourself and anyone you are caring for. Perhaps this is what makes caregiving so difficult, because there is a beginning and there is going to be an end, but what happens in between is un-chartable, and when exactly the end is coming is something we are not given to know, so it is difficult to make plans.

When we know as much as possible about what we are dealing with, however, that can lend us strength and stability. As caregivers, it is up to us to help comfort our loved ones and lead them safely through the strange and frightening land in which they now live.

A Few Things I Figured Out.

- It is important to realize that illness – even a minor one - changes everything. The regular rules no longer apply.

Experiencing or helping someone through an illness will be different from anything you've experienced before. This is a frightening occurrence for everyone involved and we need to be gentle with ourselves and our loved ones. Respect and empathize with the fact that they may try to hide or deny their symptoms. If you have ever been ill and felt the ways the body can betray itself as I have, you will have at least some idea of how this feels. Emotions and emotional states like fear, anger, frustration, denial, and depression are common accompaniments to illness in general and dementia in particular because there is a loss of control, autonomy, and self-worth - a loss that will be felt both by sufferer and by caregiver.

- People with illness often feel abandoned, disenfranchised and without. Make your loved one feel that they still matter by paying attention to them, being close and touching are all good ways of showing a person that he is loved, cared for, and safe. When you touch an ailing person, you are saying, "You are not alone – I am here." Even though dementia steals memories, and personalities, and abilities, it doesn't steal away what makes us human. We have human souls in our care and they want to continue to feel necessary and of value. You can never get it perfect or exactly right. It takes great effort to keep your loved ones autonomous and to provide the most dignified and loving care. Allowing them to feel as if they exist and are being listened to is vital. Maintain intimacy and some quality of life: sensory experiences that are pleasing include - good food, sun, comfortable chairs, music, soft fabrics, lotions or fragrances.

- There are new challenges to be navigated in this country like medical care, health and housing choices, finances, and feelings about illness. I had some experience with it because of my chronic condition but others may not; believe me when I say, entering the medical domain is like nothing else. Expect the best and prepare for the worst became my motto; keep good records, write things down, have contingency plans, and do research beforehand into medical procedures, housing options, in-home care, disease progression and possible diagnoses because, as I learned, diagnoses and needs can change!

- Educate yourself and others on the dementia syndromes. Advocate for your loved ones and other sufferers; you are the first line of understanding and defense for your care-taker. Normalize what dementia sufferers are going through and how others see them. You are their face to the world and the filter of the world's input. There are many ways to help change societal attitudes toward dementia, including learning the facts of the disease, avoiding making light of the condition, and maintaining relationships with people with dementia, especially as the disease progresses.

- Be aware of what input and stimuli is entering your care receiver's environment. Assess whether television, radio, conversations or other stimuli are distressing or agitating them. Make sure their environment is calm, peaceful, and comforting. Limit loud or unnecessary input. "Sundowning" is now an accepted physical phenomenon that more caregivers and facilities are becoming aware of. In the late afternoon, sufferers can become agitated, confused, upset, or comatose - or may act out violently. There are techniques for calming and redirecting behavior – medications are usually not necessary.

- Caregiving, by necessity, becomes about the moments – crazy and otherwise. Good times, jokes remembered, times together, mini catastrophes, shared struggles - all micro occasions and crazy junctures that punctuate what is a long, slow journey. By their very nature, these moments define the act of caregiving. It is these times and experiences that color and give dimension to our lives together.

- As caregivers, we hold everything - the moments of beauty and disappointment, joy and sorrow, introspection and companionship, horror and loss, spirit and feeling - for our loved ones, and we always will. We hold their humanity for them, and we increase our own, through our caring and our service, and our authenticity. This is very often a stupid, dirty, thankless, challenging, frustrating, and heart-breaking job – and yet, we can make it matter. We can make it mean something.

6.

Sibling Rivalry.

"Our siblings push buttons that cast us in roles we felt sure we had let go of long ago - the baby, the peacekeeper, the caretaker, the avoider.... It doesn't seem to matter how much time has elapsed or how far we've traveled." - Jane Mersky Leder

Although there was no big fight or defining estranging event, my sister and I don't have much of a relationship with each other. I am not always sure exactly why, although I have some suspicions. I realized after years of therapy that *none* of the members of our family really knew how to be in relationship with each other. Every relationship between the members of my family was a surface one.

As children, my sibling and I tolerated each other and were allies against our parents. I remember many shared moments, fun experiences, games, and even confidences and supportive times. There are still random phrases and words which can, when mentioned by one of us to the other out of the blue, spark strong shared memories of events or aspects of our childhood. As young adults, we were close, sharing each other's lives to a certain extent, and supporting each other through difficult times, like the death of our mother.

Together, we lived through our difficult religious upbringing and the shame and fear around illness, although it scarred us for all time in different ways and we developed very different coping mechanisms. I developed rheumatoid arthritis when I was twenty-one. Unfortunately, my sister shares my father's biological tendency toward depression, which I didn't really realize fully until my early thirties. That depression escalated into debilitating anxiety issues and panic attacks.

In our late twenties and early thirties, we were both single and we spent time together, sharing our fears and dreams. For me, this was a nice time of companionship and bonding. Then, of course, my father's illness intruded. Suddenly, we had the immense pressure of family crisis and obligation on our relationship. Our father's dementia definitely signaled the beginning of the end of whatever relationship we may have had.

During the first few months we were taking charge of my father and his affairs, when everything was chaotic and shocking, I was struggling with a great anger about my father's needs versus my own. He had not cared for me and I was resistant to caring for him. My sister was strong and capable and she took charge, for a while at least. After a few months, I rejoined her and took up my share of the care burdens. Together we were able to get things organized and moving.

After the crisis, she began to fade out of the picture more and more and I began to assume greater and greater responsibility. When I knew I was going to move in with Dad, I tried to rely on her for support, inviting her over for dinner and to watch movies - invitations she never accepted. She would help me with the bigger financial and clerical decisions, but I definitely became responsible for the day-to-day work of caring for our father.

I don't write much about her now, both because I try to respect her privacy and also because I'm living and writing about <u>my</u> story – her story and her experiences are largely her own to tell.

When I do write about her, I struggle to do so fairly. In fact, I did write about her in my first book, albeit trying to present as fair and unbiased a picture of events as possible, including my own issues, patterns, and petty feelings.

While I know a little about *how* she thinks and what it is that may influence her actions, I don't know her well enough anymore to know *what* she thinks or feels about Dad, her life, me, or anything else. I would not now presume to know what she needs or hopes for, or even what she wants from her life. We are connected only through Dad, and that tentatively. It would be a lie, however, to say that her actions haven't affected me in my caregiver journey and that I don't have my share of hard feelings.

We have not always been able to see eye to eye about Dad, his care and needs, and our responsibilities in response to them. In this we are no different from many other families, apparently, and it has caused us our share of problems. It definitely made caring for Dad difficult; her capriciousness towards him, his care, and me. Her level of involvement fluctuated monthly: one month she would claim to want to be involved while the next she would say that she was "pretty much done with Dad" or, "Didn't want to be involved in his daily care and feeding."

In the whole time of my stay in Dad's house, she rarely visited or spent time with Dad, or me, and it both frustrated me and made me sad. I felt a profound pity for what she was missing and would never be able to get back. He was slipping away little by little and she seemed to be in denial about it. It annoyed me that there was so much to do and I was getting so little help from her, even though she lived fifteen minutes away from me and Dad. Even worse, she seemed to be under the impression that she was doing more than she really was – or at least that's how it seemed to me. Her argument against doing more was that my reasons for caring for Dad were not hers – that she didn't have the same feelings of affection or duty – and didn't feel the obligation to care for him. I couldn't deny the truth of this, nor could I compel her to visit him – it wasn't really my place to force a détente between them.

After I had lived with Dad as his caregiver for a year and a half, I received a call from her, informing me that she had bought a house in another state. We had just started to talk about assisted living facilities for Dad, including how to go about finding a good one, and when we should get the whole process started. It was going to be a long, complicated, and emotional job.

For a while, I had hoped that even with all of our problems and expectations of each other, and her desire to distance herself from our Father, she would somehow come around and be there. But there didn't seem much chance of that happening from a different state. I could see now the extent to which she would go to get away from all expectation and responsibility and filial connection. Even if she eventually moved back to where we lived, the reality would most likely remain the same – she just didn't want to be involved. I realized I was truly alone.

*

In a study of women caring for parents with dementia, sibling discord was cited as the most common, and wearing, form of stress. It is one of the main issues of family caregiving (note the word, family, which many would say was the whole problem right there) and it is the single most common family complaint I've encountered – personally and professionally.

I know exactly what it is like to be aggravated, abandoned, and antagonized by a sibling when in a caregiving situation. Siblings are often the very best at knowing our weaknesses and triggers and exploiting them, just as we can be very knowledgeable about theirs. Siblings can both understand and hurt each other more acutely than almost anyone else. Most families build complicated internal emotional structures with each member taking part.

Within a family, each member will usually assume a particular role; "the Black Sheep", "the Pretty or Smart One", "the Rule Follower", "the Peace-maker", "the Baby", etc. These roles become accepted and ingrained within a family, regardless of how inappropriate or out of date they may become, and can be difficult to shake. We can find ourselves continuing to act out these roles while around our family, even if we have managed to drop them in our private lives.

Sibling relationships can be as difficult as the ones we have with our parents – sometimes even more so. We all have feelings, expectations, resentments, disappointments, and perceptions connected to, aimed at, and in relation to, our siblings. Birth order, age, number of years apart, relationships with and/or similarities with each parent – all of these things contribute to different experiences.

Siblings are usually from different generations, and may have been shaped in different ways by beliefs and experiences. Each sibling will have had a different experience within the family – as a child and as an adult. Two siblings can't have had exactly the same childhood, even in the same family. Even when close in age, they will have their own memories and feelings around childhood and shared parents, and they may have their own motivations and blind spots when it comes to family. It can be difficult to truly know what your sibling believes happened or didn't happen in the past, or how they have been shaped by the same people and events that shaped you. It is also difficult to know what they're feeling about current family events.

Older siblings may feel they had too much responsibility in the care of younger siblings, or may resent perceived inequalities in affection, freedoms, and material possessions. It can be difficult for an older sibling to accept that a younger sibling has grown up and changed and must be taken seriously. The rank provided by age or birth position can be a hard one to give up. Younger siblings may feel they lived in the shadow of older children, or didn't get as much attention.

Younger siblings may have also, consciously or unconsciously, regarded older siblings as surrogate parents or authority figures, sparking needs and expectations that may be difficult for the older sibling to fulfill. Resentment and other difficult feelings at these expectations and failures can arise in both individuals. Like parents, siblings will never be who we needed them to be in the past and they will never be exactly what we need them to be in the present.

The family hierarchy can be incredibly challenging to navigate and overcome. I can say with utter familiarity that it is extremely difficult as a younger sibling to escape years of oppression and subordination to an elder sibling and stand up for yourself and your rights. You may still feel like the younger, stupider, inferior youngster. You may still feel as if you have to prove yourself, and defend yourself, and protect yourself against the potential scorn and superiority of an older sibling – even one who has taken little to no responsibility.

This is true even if you have, in true super-hero fashion, competently taken charge, arranged and managed beautifully the complex life of your care receiver, as well as your own. No matter how mature and competent you are alone, you may still find it incredibly difficult to break out of old roles and patterns whenever you are together. In short, in a cruel twist of fate, you will always be the little sister or brother – even when you are both in your seventies and one of you is on oxygen and the other in a wheelchair.

Of course, you don't have to be caring for an ill parent to have a poor relationship with a sibling highlighted, but a stressful or crisis situation does tend to bring it to the fore. The illness of a family member appears to be one of the most challenging situations a family can face. There is something about the demands of caregiving on a family that tends to shake things up and mercilessly exposes, and acts on, the family fault lines; roles and assumptions, money, health, acceptance and repression.

*

Intellectually, I have always understood why my sister finds it so difficult to have anything to do with our Father. After all, we were raised by the same man! I know that she shared many of the same issues with Dad and our upbringing that I did. However, I also know that she and my father had a more difficult relationship in many ways than the one that he and I shared. They found it very difficult to relate to each other, although I know he yearned to be close to her – he just didn't know how. In many ways, she had to seclude herself from him to protect herself, and I understood that.

So, like me, you may not wonder *why* a sibling, for example, isn't present in the caregiving – like me, you probably already know or can guess. However, you may spend a lot of time wondering *how* they manage it. How are they able to so neatly sever themselves from duty, responsibility, and family commitment? You may often wonder, as I do, what they are thinking or planning or feeling about the whole thing, and when the situation may change, and how.

What I really don't know is *how* my sister was able to decide not to be involved. Did she just turn off those parts of her heart and brain, or does she just not possess them? Is she just one of those people who don't know how to care? I don't know how much thought my sister has given to Dad and his illness - especially as he has gotten worse. I don't know whether she realized the full truth of the situation and didn't care. She may have been in complete denial about his illness and prognosis or she may have been grieving about it and about his eventual loss. Either way, it hurt that she couldn't bring herself to be more involved.

What is also very difficult for me, even now and keeping in mind that it might be petty, is how my sister may interpret and explain her role in Dad's life to others. It is still hard for me not to think about and resent what she might be saying to other people in her life about Dad and about me. I have often felt that, in many ways, she was an emotional tourist, and that she has been experiencing this journey with Dad through me.

When she used to ask me how Dad was, what he was doing or feeling, or for details of his care, I was reluctant to say too much. I worried that she took what I told her about Dad and used it to make other people believe she was involved as much as I was; retelling the story in a certain way to make herself look better. I used to think a lot about how she might be spinning the situation, and the fact that she could be saying anything, telling any tale, and not only could I not control it, but I wouldn't even know for sure she was doing it! Whether any of this is fair or even rational is up for debate; the reality is that it made me angry – it still does, although I've learned ways to deal with it.

Eventually, with a lot of emotional soul searching and therapeutic help, I was able to take a step back and gain some perspective. There would never be any way to control what she said or did or thought. I cannot control the stories she tells to other people, or the stories she tells herself, or the ways she spins the situation. I may want to but I can't.

Another thing that made the whole situation more irritating was that Dad still seemed to prefer her to me, even though I was the one doing all the work and making all the sacrifices. It used to make me angry and despondent when dad would ask about my sister after I had just spent hours of my life making *his* life comfortable. It broke my heart when my dad asked how my sister was doing, or whether I'd seen her. I was angry with her for her perceived abandonment of us; sometimes I even tried to convince or bribe her to visit.

I have read similar stories from other caregivers – they are the ones constantly present, but the parent yearns for the inaccessible sibling. It can be completely crazy-making to have given hours of your time and energy to cooking and cleaning and caring for your loved one, only to watch them want something, or someone, different. It becomes extra difficult when trying to manage or assuage the feelings of your care receiver about the great hole left by your sibling.

My friend who has just become a caregiver has a brother in another state who has *flirted* with helping out; darting forwards coyly with good intentions only to retreat in fear and bluster. She tried to contact him during her mother's latest, serious, illness, only to be rebuffed. She had to then help her mother with the bewilderment and heartbreak of his inexplicable actions.

People fume and fret, feel guilty and feel sad for their parent, who, of course, misses and constantly asks after the prodigal child. I read one woman's blog posting about the subject. She seemed like a wonderful caregiver, who visited her mother daily, did all sorts of chores and nice things for her, and had virtually put her life on hold for her mother; yet all her mother could do was talk about this woman's brother and how great he was and how he never came to see her.

On the one hand, this woman loved her mother, and it broke her heart to see her mother disappointed, but she also felt huge rage and frustration for her brother's lack of caring and lack of willingness to make any sacrifices. She was also angry at her mother for continuing to prefer the brother. It's exhausting to hold these two powerfully conflicting emotions about family, yet it's something caregivers experience all the time. It's exhausting trying to manage everyone's expectations and their actions and reactions. And that's exactly the point – you can't control them anymore than you can control the seasons or the tide. People act and react according to the feelings and event of the moment, colored always by the experiences of the past.

I've seen caregivers driven crazy purely because they cannot control what their sibling is doing – or not doing. They are doing what they are doing because of who they are, not because they weren't *aware* of the entirety of the situation. Trying to change a family member can be a lot like spitting in the ocean and expecting to raise the water level. Your siblings are probably going to do exactly what they are going to do, help out exactly as much as they are going to help, according to their own ideas, childhood experiences, belief systems, and feelings. A sibling will act selfishly because they have *always* been selfish, or will be difficult and bossy because that's how they've always been.

Again, they aren't the person we can change, effect, help, act on, etc. – w*e* are. As difficult as it may be, we have to let go of our past and present expectations and allow our siblings to meet us however they can. We must remind ourselves that they will be who they are and do as much or as little as they can, regardless of how much we struggle and complain. The person we must really work on is ourselves. The only person you can control is *you* – and I know it can be a frustrating cliché but it really is the only strategy that will absolutely work.

There will always be things about your siblings that bother you. Let it go. You can't control whether they act like a jerk, but you can control how you react. You can't manage their actions, but you can manage your response to them. You cannot direct what they say to others or how they present or portray a situation – it is a physical and emotional impossibility. What you can manage is your behavior - your actions - the ways in which you are doing vital and admirable work for your loved one, the knowledge that you are doing the right thing for you at this time in caring for your loved one, the honesty about caring for yourself and asking for respite, the awareness that you are managing your own feelings and working through them. This is powerful stuff, and it is all for you.

Unfortunately, this also means that you can't control the actions, reactions, and emotions of your care receiver. This means not only that they have to experience whatever feelings they are going to experience as a result of your siblings' actions, but that you have to *watch* them experience it, and let it happen. You can't force your sibling to act and you can't take your care receiver's pain away.

I know that you don't want such pain to be inflicted on them. In fact, this is probably why you are giving care, because you don't want them to be hurt and you want the best for them. This can be the toughest thing of all and there's no way around it if you are going to avoid being driven crazy. But ultimately it is good practice for listening to yourself and your needs, giving good, emotionally healthy, care, and setting boundaries.

Admittedly, this is a difficult place to be in. We have enough to deal with as caregivers, without having to navigate complicated emotional minefields with our family members. It is tempting to blow them off – or let them blow us off – and be content to nurture our bad feelings. It is tempting to be a martyr and a victim – believe me, I've been there – but it is also inefficient and exhausting.

The only person who is marinating in this potent brew of negativity and resentment is you. They are probably completely unaware and unaffected. So finding your voice as a caregiver and member of a challenging family is probably the best thing you'll ever do and the best weapon you'll ever have. Open up and start talking about the realities of the situation and your feelings.

Speaking up to your sibling(s), regardless of their reaction, is for you. Speaking your truth about the situation and your feelings is for you. Give it some thought and then take responsibility for anything that is coming from you – take responsibility for your part in the dynamic because there are always two sides. This is your truth, these are your feelings and they can't dispute them – they are valid. The only drawback is that your siblings' feelings are valid, too, they will have their own truth and it may be different from yours. It may be so different that it makes you angry, however, it is still valid.

And one of the real beauties of opening yourself up and putting your truth out there is that you create the possibility for change – even if it is tiny. Perhaps your sibling didn't know how you were feeling - now they can change their behavior or their actions because they have correct information. It can seem as if something is so obvious to us, however, we may not be aware how good we are at hiding it or keeping it quiet. I am particularly good at this – I think I am yelling (metaphorically) about something when in actuality I am barely whispering.

Perhaps taking responsibility for your own feelings will make them think about their feelings. You will have been as honest as possible: you won't have employed guilt tactics; you won't have hidden behind passive aggression (at least as much as possible); and you will have owned up to your own issues. Maybe they will feel more inclined to help you in some small way. I also know that it's possible they won't really respond to what you have to say, which is the killer catch-22. The point is, you have made some space. You have bravely cleared out years of emotional clutter and old belief systems. Who knows what will grow there in its place?

I ultimately realized that I had to stop focusing on my sibling and what she was doing, and just focus on myself. I had to take charge of, and work through, my own feelings - grief, abandonment, self-righteousness and martyrdom, among others - and not let them color the situation. Most importantly, I had to start dealing with my sibling and her faults as is, not as the person I wanted or needed her to be, in just the same way I had come to terms with my father.

I had to let go of my expectations, acknowledge she would never be the sister I wanted or needed, and set my own boundaries. I had to allow her to deal with Dad in her own way, just as I was doing, and stop trying to control everything. Eventually, I realized something that either nobody thinks about, or nobody admits to, and that is that there are certain perks to going it alone.

*

I came to realize that I preferred the situation the way it was, with my sister not participating. Not only because it was simpler, but because I could have everything my way, and do things exactly how I wanted to. I am a person who likes a certain amount of control, and I realized that even though I had relinquished control over my sibling and her situation, I still had quite a bit of control over my father's. I can manage his care pretty much exactly as I choose. I can make decisions and choices according to my knowledge of Dad and his needs, without having to negotiate or compromise. You can get a lot done when you're not in a committee.

Although her lack of involvement still bothers me occasionally, I have mostly come to terms with it and with what she is able to do. I have discovered that she is an excellent sprinter, but a lousy marathoner. Interestingly, her skills lie in managing a short-term crisis, and mine lie in dealing with the long haul. I should have known this, actually, knowing what I do of how she operates. She has always functioned best in crisis and urgency: school papers finished at the last moment; work projects completed on, or a little past, deadline; huge decisions (like moving to another state) made spontaneously.

Several times, there has been some emergency with my father that I have been unable to deal with because I was ill or out of town or something. In those few cases, I have called on my sibling to take over, which she has done quite capably for a brief time, dealing with the problem in the short term until I was able to take over again. Then it becomes my job to pick up Dad's care and handle the event for the duration while she fades back into the background. In these instances, I've been able to *take* care when I needed it in the only way that my sibling could give it.

I know that I will probably never stop pondering, and, let's face it, being frustrated by, the whys and wherefores of my sibling, and the reasons she did what she did and does what she does. I will probably continue to feel a range of emotions, from resentful and irritated to compassionate and patient. It is likely that the situation will never fully resolve. Now, even though we live in the same city, we have drifted apart, seeing each other generally once a year at Christmas and exchanging the occasional email saying we should get together.

We started out as a small family, and someday soon my dad will die, leaving just the two of us. This quiet planet around which we orbit will be gone, along with its pull of family gravity. I fear that at that point - the moment of his passing - we will cease altogether to exist as a family, and we will drift apart into our own lives. I'm not sure I would change that if I could; I think I've finally come to terms with how things are, and likely to be.

A Few Things I Figured Out.

- Sibling relationships, like all family relationships, are difficult and fraught with peril. The burdens of illness and caregiving often only make them worse. This is when fault lines appear and people's characters, and old fears and resentments, surface. Your sibling may act in ways that are completely inexplicable to you, that cause you great grief and frustration. You are not alone, however! There are hundreds of forum threads, Facebook groups, blogs, and books full of sibling stories and the difficulties caregivers have gone through when dealing with them. There are people venting everyday about the same problems you are having!

- I have managed to forgive many things, although I doubt I will ever forget. And that's really all I'm saying; no one's asking you to forget, or even to forgive, but only to explore the events and your feelings, and decide what you are able to do from there. Remember that we can only control ourselves, and that imperfectly, and that no one can go back and change the past. It can be easy to understand the situation and our siblings' motivations intellectually yet still feel compromised emotionally, which is why having someone to help you navigate the whole thing is so helpful. I don't know what I would have done without my therapist as my sounding board, shoulder to cry on, and benchmark for what is "normal."

- I know how nice it would be to get some recognition of the sacrifices we make and the effort we put into caring for our loved one. I can't remember the last time my sister said thank you, or even acknowledged the work I do. It is human nature to want to be appreciated, especially when we feel like we are making superhuman sacrifices and doing good work. We just want to be recognized; is that so wrong? We don't need a psychological breakthrough, an epiphany, or an abasement. We may not even need a thank you, but what we would like is acknowledgment. —I see you. —I see that you are doing what I cannot or will not do. Unfortunately, you may have to come to terms with the fact that you might never hear it, however – at least from them. There are probably plenty of other people saying it to you, so try to listen to them.

- Why are we so hesitant to speak our truth, to make them understand? I know it's often because of past issues but we are adults now. I think it is up to us to practice speaking up and making ourselves heard. Perhaps much of my resentment and hard feelings could have been avoided if I'd been a little bit better about communicating my feelings and expectations. Maybe it would have helped if we'd sat down and gone through a list of present and future responsibilities and issues and decided who could and should do what. (Like the expectation that nobody was going to move out of state!) If I'd had something written down that we'd both agreed to, perhaps I would have felt I had more control or more recourse when things began to devolve onto me.

- It's a reality in this world that some people are just really good sprinters, but are not good in a marathon. Sometimes it can be just that easy – finding out what people are good at and having them do it. If one sibling lives far away but is good with money, for instance, have them balance the check book and pay bills. If a sibling can't face spending time with your care receiver, have that person do the laundry or grocery-shopping so that you don't have to. I have learned how to *manage* our sibling situation, and my feelings about it, to a certain extent. I have learned how to exist with the situation as it is, not how I would wish it to be.

7.

Home Sweet Home.

"Home is the place where, when you have to go there, they have to take you in."
Robert Frost

I tentatively pushed open the door of Dad's room, a place I usually tried not to enter since I knew Dad liked his privacy and didn't like things in his room to move. I don't know why I was so apprehensive since Dad wasn't even in the house. I had arranged for Del to take him out all day for two days in a row so I could perform the difficult task I was there to do: pack up my dad's clothes and as much of his most important stuff as I could without him noticing. He didn't know it, but this would be his last night in the house. I was secretly moving him to Assisted Living the next day.

Amazingly, I pulled it off, managing that first day to keep the room looking as it always had - piled up with clothes, dusty books, soft drink cups, and other flotsam – even after packing a few boxes and suitcases of clothing and other items. The second day, minutes after Dad and Del left, the movers came for the furniture and boxes, taking them over to the new apartment where we were all waiting to put it all in place.

My boyfriend at the time, Charlie, and I worked frantically to unpack clothes, hang pictures, put together and make the bed, and do our best to make it feel like home. We brought Dad's cat over and installed him in the new apartment, then waited for Del to bring Dad to the facility where we were all to meet, ostensibly for dinner.

We enjoyed a very nice dinner in the dining room, then took dad up to his new apartment and showed him around. We sat him down and told him that this was now his home: he would be living here because it was more comfortable and safe. He was angry and confused, but there was nothing he could do, so he sat there, a terrible frown on his face.

After an uncomfortable hour, we left him with Del, who would stay with him in the room overnight, and the cat and drove tiredly home. It had been a difficult two days. And while I didn't feel proud of sneaking around, deceiving and blindsiding my dad, and leaving him in a place I knew he hated – I also knew it was the right thing to do for both of us.

*

Choices about Dad's care were consistently difficult: the progression of his disease often made it a challenge to fit him into any of the options that I had available to me. His dementia presented in such strange ways - taking some faculties but not all, leaving him capable and aware in some areas but not in others.

He was very fit and strong physically but couldn't take care of himself or make complex decisions and he was also paranoid and in denial. At times, I had to kind of shoehorn him into a situation that fit some needs but not all of them. There were never perfect solutions but I made the best decisions I could, using my imagination and whatever resources were available.

Finding some sort of Assisted Living or Memory Care facility was always part of the plan. I knew I would be able to be his direct caregiver for the first few years of his illness, but I knew that as his illness progressed, there would come a time when I would have to move him out of his own home, as wrenching as that would be, and into a facility where he could get exactly the care that he needed. This was not a reality that was ever going to change; his illness was going to get worse, and I couldn't care for him.

I had my own chronic illness to deal with that reduced my abilities and energy-level, and that I did not want to aggravate. I knew that there was no way I would be able to perform some of the physical tasks that are the reality of caring for someone that is disabled. I knew I would not be able to lift him on and off the toilet or out of a chair, help him stand or walk, catch him if he fell, or restrain him during an aggressive or delusional episode. I would also be unable to perform all the chores of housekeeping while at the same time attending to his hourly needs, nor would I have the stamina to sustain sleepless nights as he wandered or needed attention.

Even more importantly, I knew that, emotionally, there was no way I could perform personal and intimate tasks for my father like bathing and toileting or changing diapers; there were some lines I couldn't, and wouldn't, cross. For some caregivers, these tasks are no different from any other they perform and are just another way to show their love for, and service to, their charge. Others are uncomfortable with these tasks due to modesty, because they are too personal or feel disrespectful, or because the emotional relationship they had with their charge does not allow for this kind of intimacy.

This was the case for me. Although I was watching him lose his faculties, both physically and mentally, I didn't want to lose everything about him. I wanted to sustain a certain distance and respect for him as my father, and keep him in that place in my mind. There were certain boundaries I refused to cross.

As I approached two years of being Dad's caregiver, I knew that the time had come to make a move, not only for his well-being but for mine. When I was at his house, I was cooking, cleaning, shopping, and looking after him. When I was not with him, I was still spending a fair amount of time handling his affairs and coordinating his aides and activities. I was starting to wonder if this was all my future was going to hold. And it could be really, really boring being a housewife all the time, answering the same questions over and over, and trying to keep him entertained.

I tried to take him out and about every day I was with him so that he didn't get bored, however, I was starting to run out of places to go. It was also stressful riding herd on my dad when we were out; I was always worried he was going to wander off when I was in the restroom, or that I would somehow lose track of him. I was also afraid of his disease changing and getting worse, or that he would do something to jeopardize his health and safety or damage the house.

In fact, I was actually afraid of the house itself. It was not in the best repair and I worried that it could flood or catch on fire, although honestly, it was so full of mildew that it would probably not have burned. When I was home, I was always half-listening for the phone and when it did ring, I was apprehensive about what I was about to hear.

Most importantly, I wanted to move him while he was still somewhat lucid and able to make the shift to a new home. Opinions are divided about when it is best to move people with dementia but it seemed best to me that he be able to recognize his new surroundings. It just seemed the time had come to change directions with Dad's care – which was what led us to the Assisted Living Facility.

*

In the past, caregiving was performed at home, by family members. People didn't live as long with their illnesses, however, so care was not required for the extended periods of time we are seeing today. Improvements in medical technology mean people are living longer, and living longer with chronic illnesses that take a lot of care. Societal and family changes have also taken place that affect caregiving.

More people work outside the home than ever before, and it is generally an accepted fact that two incomes are needed to live comfortably. Families are more separated, living greater distances from each other – making it difficult to provide care. It is true that a lot of caregiving is still performed in the home by family members - more than 70% of Alzheimer's sufferers currently live at home. However, for many families it is longer feasible or possible to personally provide care in the home to a loved one.

We would all like to believe that only we can provide the best care for our loved ones, but that's simply not always the case; sometimes, other choices are more appropriate. Sometimes we physically can't provide care, or we can't do it all alone and need care assistance, or a facility will offer better exposure to friends, activities, and other socializing opportunities. Being responsible for someone who needs a high level of care is a huge challenge, and there are no easy answers.

The reality is that there are no perfect options – there is no one solution that is better than all the others. The choice of who will care for your loved one is the most important, and difficult, one of all because there are so many different types of care, and so many different places and people who can provide it. The fact that many different care options are now available is a good thing: the difficulties begin when people try to make judgments on how and where care is given. Attempting to establish what is the best thing, the right thing, or the normal thing to do is impossible and I am here to tell you there is no such place as "normal."

Odds are good that this is a completely new situation for everyone involved. Few of us are familiar with these types of decisions on how and where to provide care and who will do it. Any choice we make about who is to care for our loved one, and where that care will take place, will have its own benefits and drawbacks, its own strengths and weaknesses - without exception.

Decisions on institutionalized care must be made according to the needs of each individual and family, and according to the details of each situation. They must take into account not only the best interest of the care receiver, but also the best interest of the primary caregiver and the family. Care choices made due to guilt, family pressure, or shame, can ultimately prove harmful to caregivers who haven't been able to make their needs heard. They can also potentially prove harmful to the care receiver if they aren't the most appropriate choice.

Everyone seems to have an opinion, pitting facilities against in-home care with an aide, against in-home care by the family. It can be a contentious, hotly-argued issue, with each person thinking *their* way of thinking is the right way. Some point to abuse in facilities as an argument for homecare only, yet statistically, elder abuse occurs most often by relatives of the elder. Others point to family care being more personal and one-on-one, with better response times and options. And yet, many accidents occur at home, and not all family caregivers are good ones.

A recent study said that more than ½ of the care receivers cared for at home had inadequate meaningful daily activities. Another Johns Hopkins study stated that most family caregivers have multiple unmet needs, including lack of access to resources and referrals to support services and education on how to care. At-home care, provided by family, isn't always the best way to go. I would argue strongly that, regardless of what anyone says, there is no right way when it comes to where care is given and who gives it.

Keep in mind that giving care at home, by necessity, changes the relationship between those involved: from spouses to caregiver and care receiver; from parent and adult child to person needing care and person giving it. It can be hard to get past new duties, attitudes, and expectations to the old relationships. Placing a care receiver in a facility means that they will get their care from a paid professional, and the family caregiver can go back to just being a spouse or daughter. A relationship not based on caregiving can be retained. One woman I spoke to said that as soon as she placed her husband, she could see him as her husband again, and some part of their former loving relationship resurfaced, without the duties and aggravations of giving care. Don't underestimate the emotional benefit of this. In the end, home-care and facility-care both have their strengths and weaknesses, positives and negatives.

*

There are many ways to be of service to our loved ones other than personally giving care. Some people who have enough money to hire full-time caregivers may feel guilty when hearing the stories of other, less-fortunate families who are run ragged providing care. There is nothing to feel guilty about in this situation; it is a blessing to have enough to provide for your loved ones, and to have the energy to be fully present with them.

Other people will always have opinions about what we choose, just as we will question and second-guess our *own* choices. Looking back on it now, I'm sure many people judged the decisions I made according to their own standards of behavior and rightness. Even *I* sometimes had doubts about the decisions I was making; the only way forward was just to keep doing the best I could; keep reminding myself that I couldn't control everything; and change whatever wasn't working.

I was confident that when looking at facilities - what can be a long and laborious process - I could find one that would do the best job possible. Fortunately, my dad had had enough foresight when he was lucid to provide for himself financially, which would also help in my choice. I decided that an Assisted Living Facility with an attached Dementia wing suited his needs the best and I toured a lot of them. As I toured facilities all over our area, I asked as many questions as I could think of about the care staff, about procedures, care styles, and facility rules.

I inquired what their policies were about allowing a resident to "be" where and when they were in time and in their minds. I asked whether sexual relations were permissible between residents, since I knew it was a possibility that Dad could meet and develop a relationship with another resident. I appeared at facilities during mealtimes to check how clients were fed and what the food tasted like. I appeared at other times during the day to gauge activities and what the caregivers did with their charges. I stuck my nose in every corner to check for the smells of urine and neglect.

I was looking for a facility that had both an Assisted Living section and a dementia wing that I liked. I wanted the facility to adapt to my father's changing disease, not the other way around. I wanted a place he could potentially spend the rest of his life, thereby avoiding a confusing and disturbing move to another facility. I finally chose a very nice facility relatively near my home where I could adjust Dad's level of care according to his changing needs, fully expecting it would be his last home.

He would be able to live in an apartment at first, with just enough supervision and care that he could still feel somewhat independent, while being safe and cared for. He could be integrated into the life of the facility and get involved in outings and activities. Although I expected it wouldn't happen for several years, when Dad's disease worsened to the point that he needed a lot more care and attention, the dementia wing would be waiting right downstairs to receive him. It wasn't a perfect solution, few things are, but it was the best way I could determine to accommodate Dad's physical needs.

His emotional, social and spiritual needs were also very important, and I began to put plans in place providing for that support long before he entered the facility. Since outside aides were permitted in the facility, I planned to continue paying Del to come several days a week to spend time with Dad, take him out for meals, and take him to his church. I hired his old friend, Janet, to care for him two days a week. I would also spend a few days a week with my father, taking him out for lunch, or sitting with him in his new apartment.

In the end, I chose to move Dad secretly because I knew it would just agitate him to know too much about the move. At first, I reminded him several times that he would be moving, as the event approached, because I didn't want it to be a shock. The reaction I got, however, was not heartening. Dad couldn't remember our initial conversation about the move and his acceptance of its benefits, and he became irritated when I reminded him.

He brusquely brushed me off with the assertion that it wasn't necessary as there was nothing wrong with him. When I persisted, reminding him about his disease and the poor state of the house, he got even more immovable; it was obvious he thought I was the one who was crazy, and the only thing my protestations of truth were doing were making him anxious and angry.

There are many books and websites now that tell you how to find a good facility - what to look for, what questions to ask, what to expect, and what you should and shouldn't bring with you.

Unfortunately, few of them tell you the best way to actually *move* your loved one. In part, that is because it is such a subjective process. The disease affects everyone differently; each person has different reactions and personalities, and each person is able to take in, comprehend, and accept different levels of information. One particular plan may not work for everyone. However, there is a loose structure and some guidelines on which you can build your plan.

The main issue to consider is exactly how much they should be involved in the process. Should you consult them about when to move, or what facility to move into, or what they want to bring? Should you be honest about the financial and legal details? To determine the answers to these questions, you need to evaluate your loved one. If they are still in a cognitive place where they can comprehend what you are saying and are able to contribute – and aren't too angry about the move - then you might consider involving them in some of the smaller decisions.

Pick a facility for example, but bring them to it and ask which room they might prefer or what furniture they might want to bring from home. If they will react negatively to the move, keep as many details private as possible. If possible, find a room or apartment that resembles where they live already. I chose an apartment that mimicked the layout of Dad's bedroom at home, and set up his furniture in the same way he'd had it at home. We brought his bed and some familiar paintings and other objects so he would recognize his surroundings as much as possible. I'm sure it helped having familiar things around.

If you feel it necessary to tell your care receiver about what is coming, make sure you are not alone. Invite family or close friends or a trusted aide to be there at the same time. Consider asking your care receiver's doctor or a family pastor to help you. Focus on the good things that are to come.

Try to get the room comfortable and settled before bringing in your care receiver. If it would be easier for you and you loved one alike to use calming medication, then use it. Throughout the move, try to remain positive. This is a difficult transition – there are ways to make it easier and more comfortable – but it is difficult. Since afternoons can be difficult for dementia sufferers, try to perform the move in the morning, and have everyone congregate for lunch at the new facility.

Some facilities recommend the family not contact their loved one for a certain length of time after the move, citing ease of adjustment for the resident. I, personally, don't think much of this particular rule and probably wouldn't have picked a facility that recommended it. I'm sure that, in most cases, it works fine but I do have a friend who helped her father pick a facility like this for her mother. When they finally contacted the facility, they learned her mother had suffered a fall early in the first week of her residency and sustained a serious broken arm that went undiagnosed.

The facility neglected to contact the family and they were horrified to learn that the arm had become septic and she was being rushed to the hospital. Ultimately, my friend and her father had to say good-bye to their wife and mother in the hospital as she died an unpleasant death.

As I say, I'm sure this doesn't happen very often, and, in fact, could happen in any facility. The fact that they didn't know, however, because they weren't encouraged to call, is striking. The transition period is going to be difficult no matter what. It seems to me that the presence of family can only help ease that, not hinder it. I would make the decision whether to be in contact with your care receiver after the move yourself and not allow the facility to make it for you.

Unfortunately, Dad never felt as comfortable in his apartment as he had felt at home, which I knew was likely. He often referred to the facility as his "prison" and I could tell he didn't like it, even though it was a perfectly nice place with friendly people. When I appeared to take him out for lunch, he grew excited and animated as we left, an energy that would change to sullenness and disappointment when it became obvious I was returning him to the hated facility.

At first, I felt a natural guilt that I was leaving my loved one in a place he despised. With help, I realized that guilt is a worthless feeling; it doesn't change realities and it just wears you out. After a month or so, I noticed a marked difference in Dad's comprehension and emotional state, as if he had lost ground. I realized that towards the end of his stay in his house, he had been working really hard to keep himself together, to deny that he was getting worse. It was as if moving into a place of greater care allowed some part of him to relax that tension and release control even more, letting go of more lucidity. While I was sad to see these changes, I knew the effort it must have cost him to keep up appearances and I hoped that he at least felt well looked after in his new home.

*

After about two years in his apartment, and much sooner than I expected, we had to reassess his situation. Dad's disease had always caused him to wander; it was the wandering, of course, that led to me taking over his life. The wandering had stopped, though, after Del and I moved in with my dad, as if he no longer felt the need to look for help now that his needs were being met in his own home and he was relatively happy. After moving to the facility, though, the wandering began again, and it worried me.

He would leave his apartment and walk for miles. Off-duty caregivers were always reporting having seen him four or five miles away from the facility. Although he always returned, I didn't like him going so far away and I discussed it with the facility Director. She informed me that since he was a free, adult resident they couldn't keep him from leaving, but they did clip a sensor to him that alerted them to when he was at the front door so they could try to redirect him.

Several months later, it became even more of a problem when he began to return late and tired, complaining of having gotten lost on the way back. Del took him out walking as much as possible, but it still kept happening, until the problem finally came to a head. I received a call from the facility informing me that Dad had been outside when a caregiver tried to redirect him back inside. The caregiver reported that Dad had appeared not to recognize him and had been frightened, taking off and running past Del who had just arrived to pick him up.

Dad had run straight out into the busy street in front of the facility and had narrowly missed being hit by a car. Del had gone after him but it had been several hours until they returned. Apparently Dad had also failed to recognize Del and had run from him. I discussed it with the facility director, who was justifiably concerned for their liability, as well as for Dad's health, and it was decided that my father needed to be transferred for safety to the dementia wing.

I knew it was the right decision in terms of safety, but not in terms of Dad's emotional health - cognitively he was still well ahead of all of the dementia wing's residents. After we moved him into his new, smaller room, it was devastating to see Dad's reaction to the behaviors and people he saw around him; residents that were catatonic in corners and in the T.V. room, or wandered the corridors clutching dolls or clothes. He was still aware and lucid enough to know what he was looking at and be horrified by it. I compensated as best as I could by continuing to have Del take him out of the facility for trips and meals, and I visited several times a week. We both tried to keep his spirits up as best we could by spending as much time with him as we could.

Although the dementia wing was scrupulously clean and well-staffed, there were definitely times I was a little disappointed in the care he was receiving. Not that the caregivers were abusive or didn't care but because they had their schedules and duties to perform that didn't always fit Dad's needs. I would often find him left in front of the TV with other residents, even though he didn't seem to be interested in what was on. Meal times could also be a problem.

My father was a good eater but a *very* slow one, and someone needed to check periodically to see if he was eating. I felt the staff didn't always give him enough time to finish his entire meal since they had other duties to perform after meal times; whisking his plate away before he was quite done. Del and I both tried to make sure the nurse in charge and other caregivers knew to spend extra time with him at the table. Since none of these things posed a danger to his well-being, I was willing to keep him in the facility, with monitoring by me, and more often, Del, of any problems. I expected that, barring any problem, he would end his days there.

*

The fact that I was not the only person who cared for my father and that I placed him in a facility does not make me a bad daughter or a poor caregiver. I will be his caregiver until his death, regardless of who is performing his physical care, or where he is receiving it. I still spend as much time with him as I can, giving care and sharing my life with the person who remains.

I continue to manage his life in addition to my own - making sometimes difficult health care and financial choices. I always carry my phone with me because I am always on call - 24 hours a day, seven days a week – available to his caregivers for any question or concern. I will probably not move out of the area where I currently reside until he is gone, and his care is a factor in almost every important life decision I make. I am fortunate that we have only faced a few crises so far, but as Dad's illness progresses, I am sure a lot more time and energy will be required of me.

I could never have been his only caregiver - physically or emotionally. My father would have suffered from my limitations, and he wouldn't have had the benefits of others caring for him. If I had been Dad's only caregiver, he would not have had Del in his life, with all the socialization and friendship and new activities that Del brought. Del became part of the family, trusted and indispensable, and Dad's biggest advocate. Del was meant to be in Dad's life; in fact, he *changed* Dad's life.

Never underestimate the benefits that other people can bring to your loved one's life. Also, be aware that every care situation is different and you must make choices that are appropriate to you, your family, and your care receiver.

A Few Things I Figured Out.

- Some caregivers are unable for health, financial, or other personal reasons to provide care personally, and have placed their charge in a carefully picked facility where they can get the aid they need. There can sometimes be a prejudice that the only loving or "right" care is home care, but that is far from the truth – sometimes the most courageous and loving choice is knowing a facility would be better.
- Don't be afraid of considering a facility for your loved one, despite any horror stories you may hear in the media. There are as many wonderful facilities as there are terrible ones. A facility can provide things that being at home cannot, like

access to friends and activities, greater socialization, and access to round-the-clock care. There are also so many different types of care facility now that it is highly probably that you will find the perfect one for your situation and your loved one. There are many resources now designed specifically to help you find a good place; I've listed many in the Resources section.

- The most important things you can do to find a good place are simple: visit as many facilities as you can; go at different times of the day, including mealtimes so you can taste the food; assess smells, cleanliness, and how caregivers respond to residents; have a list of questions prepared and ask as many as you need to; research the caregiver-to- resident ratio and how the facility has performed for state inspections. Smaller, less over-stimulating facilities seem to work well for people with some types of dementia.

- Not every caregiver lives with or provides full-time physical care to their loved ones. All caregivers are caregivers, regardless of physical proximity or type of care given. Decide the ways you *can* be present for your loved one. Be creative. There will always be things you can do, ways you can be available and present for your loved one: read to them, sing or pray with them, groom them and rub lotion into their hands. Spouses: create moments in which your old ways of relating are recaptured, and/or find new ways. Try to connect intimately through conversation, snuggling, hand-holding, or laughing together. Our special thing was going out to lunch and for long walks, which I did with Dad every week until it was too over-stimulating for him. Now that my father can't go out I sit with him, talk to him, and read to him.

- Assisted Living is a flexible type of housing that has only existed since the late 1980's, which operates along a scale of care/need. Although residents are encouraged to be as independent as possible, it is designed for seniors needing a certain level of help with the activities of daily living, such as eating, laundry, and taking medications, but not skilled nursing. The number of Assisted Living facilities is growing rapidly, and more often than not, now includes a special wing designed for the special needs of residents with dementia. Keep in mind, Medicare does not pay for this type of care.

- Facilities have been gradually adjusting their practices in the interests of patient comfort and humanity. All the facilities I toured shared my philosophy of working *with* the dementia, some going so far as to provide mock tool benches and kitchens, dressing tables and dress-up clothes, and, memorably, a vintage car in the lobby. In fact, most places also required the family of a resident to fill out an extensive description of their life, including relationships, likes and dislikes, food preferences, hobbies, jobs, etc. so that staff could engage the resident with actual details of their past lives. I knew my dad would be just fine in the facility that I chose for exactly this reason.

- Be polite to the staff and treat them well. Food goes a long way with health care professionals – make cookies or bring treats for the caregivers. Get them on your side, and the side of your loved one. If you suspect any problems with care, arrange a meeting with the Nurse in charge and the Director of the facility. There is an unspoken understanding in facilities that residents with interested family members that visit often and are involved in their loved ones' lives receive more visits and attention and quicker care by the caregivers. Try to arrange visits or companionship as often as possible.

- Don't be afraid to advocate for your loved one, although it is best to be as tactful as possible. Abuse can be emotional, verbal, physical, sexual, and financial. If your care receiver is claiming abuse, keep calm and pay attention to what they are telling you, both verbally and physically. Listen to and soothe all of their concerns, even if you believe they are suffering from delusional thinking. It is always in everyone's best interests to discuss an incident, real or perceived, with the caregiver and a supervisor.

8.

Ex-Girlfriends Might Make Bad Caregivers.

"We are not people who touch each other carelessly; every point of contact
between us feels important, a rush of energy and relief."
— Veronica Roth, *Allegiant*

I was at home one morning, staring at a letter I really didn't
want to open – what in Harry Potter's parlance would be called a
"Howler." The envelope was lavender with a pretty paisley design –
innocuous and sweet – masking the craziness I knew was inside. The
writing on the front was scribbled and tense, and the envelope felt
thick from what was undoubtedly several pages inside. It was a letter
from Janet, Dad's friend and also one of his caregivers. It was the
latest in a very long series of notes and letters that she had been
sending me since the day she came back into Dad's life.

Dad and Janet had been in a serious relationship for several
years in the early 1990's, after my Mom died. They had met at
Boeing and she became my father's one and only girlfriend. She was
lovely, bubbly, and very friendly, and seemed like a good foil for my
serious Father. Janet was kind and very caring towards him and
although I liked her very much, she had always struck me as
emotionally needy and fragile.

Unfortunately, several tragedies had marred her life,
including the long-term disability of what seemed to be domineering
and difficult parents which required her to care for them full-time,
until they died. She had also suffered a horrifying physical attack by
a transient and was held captive in her own home over the course of
several days. The very first time we met, she told me the entire story

of this event, in what I considered a massive over-share. Although she seemed to be coping and said she was in therapy, she also seemed brittle and somewhat unfocused.

Even though at the time, I wouldn't have objected to them marrying, I wasn't sure how stable she would be in the long term. When they broke up, I asked my dad what had happened, and I got the impression that he had been unable to meet her emotional needs, and she had ended the relationship. Knowing Dad's weaknesses in that area, I wasn't surprised – I doubted he could meet a normal woman's emotional needs, and I knew hers were probably excessive.

After I became Dad's caregiver and moved in with him, Janet resurfaced and began sending cards and notes to Dad; notes I intercepted since I was dealing with all the correspondence. In the notes, she explained what she had been doing for the last several years, and asked if he would be interested in meeting up again. It was obvious that she had no idea of Dad's declining mental state and may even have been angling for the position of girlfriend once more.

I debated whether I should contact her and explain the situation, or just continue ignoring the notes. Ultimately, I decided to write back and tell her what was going on, inviting her to call me if she wanted to talk. Dad was still fairly lucid, and I was pretty sure he would remember her and enjoy a visit, but I wasn't sure how she would react to the news of his illness. She and I spoke on the phone and decided on an afternoon and a place where we could all meet for lunch. The lunch went well, although she seemed surprised and saddened by Dad's condition, but she adapted well and still treated him with kindness and care. As we all walked together after lunch she expressed the desire to see Dad more often, perhaps on a weekly basis.

Desperate to find something, or someone, to entertain Dad, I agreed. We worked out a day of the week for her to take him out to lunch and on an outing, strictly on a friendly basis. He seemed to really enjoy the time spent with her, and she reported his satisfaction in helping her fix things around her house and taking her dogs for walks. This arrangement proved beneficial for both of them and continued until the time came for Dad to move into a facility. At that point, I discussed the situation with her and asked for her assistance in helping Dad adjust to his new home. Between Del, Janet, and I, we worked out a schedule so that one of us was visiting my dad almost every day; Janet took two days, I took two, and Del took two.

Although I had balked at the idea of employing and managing any of my father's caregivers personally, preferring to work with an agency as I did with Del, it seemed fair that I pay her something for her time since it would, essentially, be her job. However, I figured that, as a competent adult and friend, she would regulate her own hours and needs. We decided that I would pay Janet a set salary, in cash, because I didn't really want to mess with time sheets that might change from week to week. She would get the same amount of money, even if she missed a day, because it would be easier for *me*. I trusted that she would either show up or stay home if sick - she didn't need to call and tell me because I didn't want to know, and I figured Dad could manage to pay her for a few sick days. I also knew she often spent more time than formally scheduled with Dad, so it all evened out.

I knew she had some physical and medical issues, and I felt it would be up to her to manage those and make decisions about what she was capable of and if she missed a day she might make it up on another day if she chose. I also explained that what she and Dad did was up to her; that she was to make her own plans and decisions, using her best judgment as to whether I needed to be alerted.

It all seemed like a fairly loose and informal arrangement would benefit everyone and I didn't anticipate any problems. I emphasized repeatedly that I didn't want to be her boss. That this was an arrangement among friends, which I was grateful for, but that I had neither the time nor the inclination to manage her. In short, I expected her to act like an adult and manage her own life, and, for a while, she did.

The facility was welcoming of both Del and Janet coming in and providing extra care. Caregiver time and energy are always tight in a facility, and the more extra private attention I could arrange for Dad was a benefit. I got the occasional call from Janet about something fun they had done or a note listing things she had observed in him, physically and mentally, which was useful for judging the diseases' progression.

She ordered special videos designed for people with dementia that included songs, little games, and views of nature – things they could watch together. She also told me about books she had read and free classes she had taken about dementia that were helping her to cope better with Dad's needs. She took him often to her house for meals or to spend time with her little dogs, which he enjoyed. She continued to let him putter around her house, making small repairs and improvements. She really seemed to be going above and beyond in her efforts.

I wondered sometimes if they were having sex, although I never asked. As far as I was concerned, she was a consenting adult and I felt Dad was still lucid enough to know his own mind in this area, especially since they had been intimate before. When I moved Dad into the facility, I had anticipated him possibly having some sort of relationship with another resident – being a still-handsome man – which was why I picked a place that had no problem with consenting sexual relationships. I figured this was roughly the same thing and I hoped they were enjoying their time together whatever they were doing.

Perhaps I should have made a different choice and made sure that a sexual relationship would be seen as inappropriate, but I made the best choice I could, based on what I observed and felt. And it seemed, at first, that the arrangement would work well. However, all too soon, the neediness and emotional fragility I observed in her ten years before began to surface. I began to receive several calls a week.

*

The calls detailed personal problems she was having, scheduling issues, what she and my father had been doing, and what she thought of the care the Assisted Living facility's caregivers were providing. She also had quite a few opinions on Del and what he was doing for my dad. It seemed as if she felt she was in competition with Del about who knew Dad best and could provide the best care.

I began to mediate between them; fielding Dels' calls about something she had done that he objected to, and assuring her that I was listening to *her* concerns about *him*. She also began trying to involve me emotionally and personally in her life, something I decidedly did not want, telling me about things she was struggling with and friends that were having problems or dying.

As I noted years before, she seemed to have problems with boundaries and what was appropriate to do and say and what wasn't, including the sharing of overly personal information. I also believe that she must have had issues with authority figures. From what she imparted to me, I knew that her mother had been an abusive, domineering figure in her life. I got the sense, as well, that she had experienced her share of insensitive and dismissive employers.

She began to project her anger, grief, and helplessness onto me by placing me in the exact role of boss/mother/authority figure that I had been trying to avoid - asking me to alternately care for and reprimand her, while resenting me at the same time. She seemed to want me to manage her life, while at the same time she fought against any hint of direction, or censure.

It took an immense amount of patience and empathy not to be triggered by her behavior and attitude, and to deal with the onslaught of needs that radiated from her. Over and over, I tried to be straightforward with her and explain the boundaries and expectations I had around the situation. I told her I trusted her with my father's safety and well-being to the point that I only needed to hear about an emergency situation. I reminded her that I was not her therapist and couldn't help her with the anger and sadness she felt about Dad's illness, or whatever issues she might be having in her personal life – that she needed to keep her personal life personal.

I reiterated that I did not want to be her employer, even though I was paying her for her time with Dad, because I considered it more as compensation to a friend for mileage, food, and entertainment provided for him. I also reminded her that I had expected from the beginning that she take full responsibility for herself and her life.

Each time she promised to comply and stop contacting me so much but nothing seemed to change. The calls increased, and letters and short notes began to appear in the mail, sometimes daily. Often, she would include some inflammatory comment or compulsive worry about Dad's well-being, or behavior, or about the facility; comments she knew I would have to respond to. At one point, she claimed that Dad seemed anorexic and anemic, that she was sure he wasn't eating properly at the facility and that his weight was dangerously low. She inferred that the caregivers and nurses might be rough with him, and that they were evasive when she tried to talk to them about him.

I trusted the facility where Dad was living and had visited there enough at unscheduled times to be fairly sure that Dad was being treated well. The caregivers appeared to be kind and competent, and there wasn't the high employee turnover that some other facilities had. Plus, I knew Del was keeping an even closer eye on the place than *I* was out of his love for Dad. While I knew that she was probably over-reacting or incorrect, comments like these always caused me to feel a little guilt and fear.

At one point, I spoke to the Director in charge of the wing to find out what she thought of Janet and whether she had been making trouble at the facility. She was very kind and told me everything was fine: that they appreciated family members that paid close attention to the care their loved ones were receiving.

Janet also began to request access to Dad's debit card, saying that it was for his benefit. According to her, he would try to pay when they went out and would be disappointed that he didn't have his card, which I had taken out of his wallet. He would tell her that he felt like a child and not an adult, and she thought having his card back would be beneficial to his mental state. There were several requests to this effect, but I refused to give her access to his card, not because I thought she would steal from him, but because the clerical and logistical ramifications seemed nightmarish. Instead, I put extra cash in Dad's wallet.

She deferred to what she called my wisdom and concern for him and his money, and stated how often he said that he loved me, yet the written missives, three and sometimes four pages long, continued. Sometimes rambling, sometimes angry and assertive, sometimes pleading, the letters kept dropping through my mailbox. And always, winding through each one, effusive sentences about how much she loved him and loved taking care of him, and how often he told her he loved her and wanted to be with her: that he had even said over and over how much he wished they were married!

The situation began to grow out of control and was taking up huge amounts of my energy. Friends urged me to fire her. I hesitated, however, because I knew she didn't make much money, and the income from caregiving helped her out. I also knew that Dad enjoyed her company a great deal and I didn't want to deprive him of that. He really liked going to her house for home-cooked meals and to perform the little home repairs he could still do. I didn't know how physical their relationship was, but I knew that he appreciated being around a woman and a friend, which probably helped him feel normal. Not for the first time, I felt caught between decisions – should I keep her on for Dad's sake, or fire her for my own.

*

The arrival of the paisley and lavender envelope took the decision right out of my hands. I had become increasingly wary of what she had to say about herself and my dad and she seemed to be getting more agitated. Her missives had become confusing and convoluted; written on all sides of each piece of paper, with several closely-written 3x5 cards inside. This particular envelope felt like the culmination of all her recent emotion and angst.

Steeling myself, I slit it open and found several pages that were almost indecipherable, they were so closely written and messy. The overall tone of the letter was one of agitation combined with manic joy. As I read the rambling sentences, I began to get more and more concerned at the crazy tone and random descriptions. Finally, I translated what I felt to be the gist of the letter, which is when the blood rushed from my head and my heart started to pound.

She detailed what a poor place she was in personally and financially; that several close friends had recently died; and that she had recently fallen off a kitchen chair into the oven door, badly striking and cutting her head. (In fact, it seemed like she was constantly and accidently hurting herself - falling over curbs and off chairs, skinning her knees, and twisting her wrists and ankles. I couldn't decide whether she was truly clumsy or whether the accidents were a cry for help and care.)

The letter continued on to say that although she had always brushed him off before, she was now seriously considering accepting Dad's last proposal. She had obviously entered into a complicated fantasy about the two of them, overlaying the current situation with their old, shared feelings, and coming to almost believe that they could have a normal relationship. She explained how much she loved him and how happy it would make her to care for him.

She gushed about "knowing" that he wanted to take care of her – that in the past he had pressed her to marry him, and promised that she would never want for anything. Several times, she reassured me that under no circumstances would she try to fight my Power of Attorney or any plans I had for Dad's care, nor would she try to come between us and his money. I would continue to be solely responsible for Dad's financial and legal affairs. She wanted only to care for him until his very last days and it would be an honor and a privilege to do so.

The first call I made was to Dad's facility, explaining as calmly as I was able the bare bones of the situation to the Director. In my panic and horror, I half expected them to tell me that Janet had picked Dad up the day before and not yet returned him. My mind jumped to what *that* phone call would sound like - Janet, raving about the lovely wedding in Vegas she and my father had just experienced!

I almost passed out with relief when the director informed me that Dad was currently playing Bingo in the Activities room. I told the Director that Janet was no longer allowed to visit my father or remove him from the premises. She assured me that they had faced this kind of situation before and that he would be safe with them.

After taking a day to have a quiet, little breakdown, and repeat loudly to my partner, Charlie, how much I didn't want to make this call, I phoned Janet. I told her that due to the distressing nature of her letter, I was concerned that she was not in a healthy place emotionally and mentally and that I thought it best that she take some time off from caregiving. I explained that for the foreseeable future, I would not be requiring her services and wished her the best.

If I thought that would mean the end of the correspondence, I was to be sorely disappointed. I continued to get cards, notes, and long letters expressing her grief at no longer seeing my father. She told me about a visit to her doctor who told her she had sustained a serious concussion during her fall in the kitchen, which explained her strange behavior. She sent long explanations about how behavioral changes are common in concussion-sufferers. She assured me that she was now fully recovered and capable of resuming her caregiving of Dad, and apologized for her lapse in judgment and sense. She repeated over and over that she would never have taken advantage of me or my father.

While I commiserated with her on her injury, I felt no desire to resume participation in the odd and troubled triangle relationship that the three of us had shared. I wasn't sure whether Dad would miss her visits or not, although I hoped it would not upset him too much, but I held firm on my decision not to let her see or care for Dad again.

With Janet, I had prolonged a poor situation out of my own inexperience and out of pity for her and respect for her feelings for Dad. I wanted Dad to keep having a meaningful connection with someone he was actually friends with, not just a paid, professional caregiver. And it did work that way, for a while. Unfortunately, it just didn't last.

*

Does this story mean that friends, romantic or otherwise, cannot give care to those with dementia? I think it depends on the situation. Friends can potentially make the *best* caregivers because of their knowledge of, and compassion for, the individual. I think it would be shame to cut them out of this role altogether. Unfortunately, it seems that we are more often trying to *encourage* our receiver's friends and colleagues to visit and be involved. Dementia can be so isolating, as people drop away out of fear, disinterest, ambivalence, or hesitance about doing or saying the wrong thing.

Some fear what they don't understand, others fear falling victim to the same fate, or that the misfortune will be somehow catching. This fear and subsequent withdrawal can be so damaging to care partners. It is exactly during the early and middle stages of illness that the distraction and affection afforded by friends can be so valuable to both the care receiver and the caregiver.

As with all things, mixing friends and caregiving depends on each person and situation. On the whole, I think this is when we need our friends the most, if only for companionship and understanding. Study after study tells us of the benefits of maintaining friendships under all circumstances; maintaining them while being a caregiver is even more important because it allows us to feel connected, cared for, and as if we have someone who is caring for *us*.

I do hear stories about care receivers whose old friends, or fellow club or association members, or work colleagues have continued to include the receiver in their weekly get-togethers, lunches, or breakfast meetings, which is so compassionate. Even though they may no longer know exactly what is going on, it gives the care receiver valuable socializing time and the feeling of still being loved.

Dad didn't have many friends; most of them had already fallen away after my mom died. Believing it was spiritually in his best interest, his church friends wouldn't have wanted to "admit" that anything was wrong with him, so none of them came to visit Dad. I did get the occasional tentative phone call, asking obliquely how he "felt." Without myself, Del, and Janet, Dad would have been alone and without friends.

Being a caregiver can be isolating, and exactly when we need our friends to rally around us. I never had anyone come visit me when I was living at Dad's, even the one or two friends who I had grown up with who *knew* Dad. I still had a few close friends, who I knew would have come in a minute if I had asked but I never wanted to bother them, and they didn't offer. We can't always blame our friends, either. Many caregivers, feeling overwhelmed or lacking in time and energy, allow friendships to drop away. Sometimes caregivers can get angry that their friends are free without responsibility, and can get on with their lives; resenting them because they aren't burdened with giving care.

If a friend is willing to take on the regular responsibility of caregiving, I think that's great, however, good boundaries are always important, as well as clear expectations of what each member of the arrangement is responsible for. I definitely tried with Janet but I think in the end, she was just too emotionally fragile to be able to sustain the work.

*

This story is also about romantic relationships: either between caregiver and care receiver, or between care receivers. This is another one of those subjects that a lot of people have opinions about when it comes up for them, but which, as a subject, is still somewhat taboo to talk about. Our society, in general, has something of a problem talking about sex; it shouldn't be surprising that sex and dementia should be even harder to talk about!

Knowing that affectionate and sexual relationships take place in facilities, I made sure that the one I placed Dad in had no problem with them. I wanted him to have as "normal" a life as possible, even while being in a facility, and if that included a relationship with another resident, that was fine. These are people living in close proximity to each other. Even though they have diminished capacity, the human instinct is to form relationships.

Sex in facilities happens a lot more than we hear about – the problems happen when it is abusive or non-consensual or between a professional caregiver and a resident. Families must make sure that, if a relationship is happening between two residents, each resident must appear comfortable with the situation. Families must also agree with each other that the situation is permissible: not all family members will be able to accept such a relationship.

Sexual relations between staff and residents is never acceptable, and there are laws, rules, and procedures to both keep it from happening, and deal with it when it does. A well-trained staff member will understand that if they are approached sexually by a resident, it usually isn't about sex, but is a reflection of some other emotion, need, or stimuli. Sometimes, a resident may be anxious about something, be desiring affection, or may have a hidden medical issue. Sexual feelings don't just go away when dementia strikes, and can be dealt with compassionately and quickly, with the right training.

Spousal caregivers that are still living with their care receiver spouses must decide what level of sexuality they still want to share. I have read posts by wife caregivers asking how to deflect demands or requests for sex from their husbands and there are various distraction techniques that can work. Explaining that it's not the right time, or that you will get to it later can work. Sometimes dementia removes physical abilities and urges from the sufferer, but they still desire affection – the demands for which may resemble sexuality. Try to maintain physical closeness through hugs or cuddling. There is an excellent book in the resource section with explanations about dementia and sexuality.

In the end, perhaps part of the problem with Janet was that they had a closer, more intimate relationship than was healthy for either of them. Janet may have been unable to emotionally distinguish between my father as he used to be and the man he had become. While I don't think that having a friend as a constant caregiver is a bad idea, it's probable that maintaining a sexual relationship at the same time is a mistake.

Every kind of care is going to have its strengths and weaknesses and you have to take the bad with the good. No care choice will ever be perfect, not even care at home by a family member; you have to find the best places, people, or situations you can and live with it. I wanted Dad to have meaningful connections with others for as long as possible as well as the best care and most enjoyable life possible. To do that, I had to trust that the people I trusted *him* with would do their best, however, there are no guarantees. Like many caregivers before me, I learned that when you are working with people, all sorts of things can happen that you have no control over.

A Few Things I Figured Out

- As my experience demonstrates, the fact that a caregiver is a friend or someone you know doesn't mean there will be no problems. However, sometimes hiring a friend of your loved one is a good solution for everyone. Make sure your boundaries are clear and firm, expectations are explained, and guidelines put down. If the emotional attachment between care receiver and potential caregiver is too strong, is inappropriate, or is causing problems, it may be best that they not give care. Above all, you must trust your instincts and gut feelings.

- Friends may not know how to react to someone with dementia. People don't want to accept that it could happen to them so they distance themselves from it as much as possible, or they may fear that they might contract it by proximity. Friends and family may stop visiting or calling the friend or family member who suffers from it because they are projecting their fears of the disease onto the individual, just don't know what to say or do, or are fearful of saying the wrong thing.

- Nurturing, human interaction is still vital, even when parts of the mind have vanished. Encouraging old friends to visit or take a care receiver out (provided they are still able) can be a great benefit for everyone involved. Maintaining your own friendships is crucial for your mental and physical well-being. If people seem like they want to be involved, don't shut them out. You may even meet new friends who share your experiences at support groups or on forums.

- Sex is still a relevant issue around dementia, facilities, and caregivers. Find out the rules and procedures in your care receiver's facility about sexual relationships between residents and residents and staff. Keep an eye on relationships between your care receiver and other residents. Keep the lines of communication open with staff and other family members. Be aware that the question of sex may come up with your own spouse, if you are their caregiver; it may just be a desire for physical affection or could be an indicator of a medical issue. Never do anything you don't want to do.

9.

They're Driving Us Crazy! And Other Problems.

"The car has become a secular sanctuary for the individual, his shrine to the self, his mobile Walden Pond." Edward McDonagh

It was the morning I went to pick up my father at his Assisted Living facility for lunch, only to find he had already been collected by a car salesman he somehow contacted, that I realized he might be having more of a problem giving up driving than I had realized. I guess I should have expected something like this to happen, considering how much he had relished driving, but I was lulled into complacency by the relative ease I'd had getting his keys when I first started caring for him.

I don't remember my father fighting me much when I took his keys, even though he loved cars and driving them. I think he had suffered a few minor fender-benders and even gotten lost a few times in the car and I think he scared himself and was willing to give up driving. Perhaps he thought it would be a temporary action, and as soon as he had proved to us that he didn't have anything wrong with him, we would give them back. And then maybe he forgot about it altogether. Although he liked being in our cars, he didn't mention driving very often or even seem upset that he couldn't drive.

As long as his aide took him out every day for long trips to different place, he seemed content. I would also take him out as often as possible, sometimes for day-long drives to state parks, just so he could feel he had truly been somewhere. He liked my little economy car, constantly asking me how the gas mileage was and how it handled. I never minded having the same conversation about my car several times a day – it was nice to see him engaged in something he liked.

After I moved him to the facility, the subject of driving resurfaced. He started talking about buying his own car – something simple with good gas mileage. It was obviously something he felt he really needed. I'm not sure whether it was the strangeness of his new surroundings that sparked this desire, or whether the idea of driving had just popped back into his head (something that happened occasionally.) I began to notice car ads and the classifieds in his apartment. Each time, I deflected him by expressing interest in his plan, asking what kinds of cars he liked, and agreeing that we could go car shopping – maybe next week. However, the desire to drive did not go away.

We had moved his Honda Del Sol to the facility so he could see it and so that Del could take him for rides in it. One morning, Del was parking his car, on the way to pick Dad up. Walking through the parking lot, he was horrified to see my father drive around the corner of the building in his zippy little car. Dad had apparently located a car key that we didn't know about in the clutter of his desk drawers. Del persuaded Dad out of the car and took the key then called me later to tell me the story. A few days after Dad's little driving adventure, I enlisted a friend to help me "steal" the car from the parking lot and drive it to my home. I sold it not long after. Dad never mentioned it again, but was apparently still thinking about a car.

Evidently unsatisfied with my slowness in obtaining him a car, he took matters into his own hands. Somehow he called a car salesman and arranged to be picked up to go car shopping. Arriving at his community that morning, I went up to his apartment, but he wasn't there. Checking the library and the on-going bingo game in the activities room, I still couldn't find him. I checked with the Activities Director, who had seen him earlier, and we tried all the familiar places again.

Becoming concerned, she took me into the Director's office and explained what was happening. It was as we once more entered the activities room, where the game was wrapping up, that one of the other residents said he had seen my father earlier - getting picked up by a young man who Dad said was from a car dealership. Could my father have arranged a pick up from a car salesman so he could buy the car he longed for? It seems he could have. (I'd never heard of this happening before, and have no idea what story he told them.)

As I frantically drove around Bellevue's new and used car lots, cursing wildly, I felt the frustration of a daughter who is still in the twilight zone between respecting a parent's continuing need for some sort of autonomy, and desiring complete control. It felt like the same problem we had experienced for so long; Dad was aware and capable in some areas, but not in other, critical, ways.

He could still act in surprising ways and achieve things I believed he was cognitively unable to do. It was still necessary to try to *influence* his behavior and actions – not control them – even though I wished I could. Dad was still a free agent as far as the community was concerned. He was still in his independent apartment within the general population, and was free to exit the facility for walks and outings.

I checked as many dealerships as I could find, hoping to stumble upon a lanky, flannel-shirt wearing, white-haired man checking out the cars. Thoughts of the havoc my father could wreak on the suburban streets on a test drive made my blood run cold. Most of the salesman were compassionate and would send someone out to search the lot but nobody had seen him.

After a few hours of fruitless searching, I returned to the facility to find that Dad had already returned. Shifty and obviously aware he had done something seriously bad, he waited for me in the lobby with the Facility Director who told me she had released the car salesman after a stern talking to. I was disappointed as I had been looking forward to having a few choice words of my own with the man, but I was not to get the opportunity.

I was both happy to see Dad unharmed - and without a new car - and furious, not unlike the parent of a naughty toddler must be after their child has wandered off at the mall. Taking Dad up to his room, I tried to explain why he couldn't drive and that what he had done was unsafe and potentially dangerous. Dad was stubborn and unrepentant in the face of my anger – in denial to the last about his condition.

I was angry and badly frightened, and irritated that he wouldn't listen to me, give me the salesman's card, or promise never to do something like this again. I felt too emotional to take him to lunch, so I explained why I was leaving and left; not without a twinge of guilt that I was both taking away something I knew he looked forward to, and ruining what had probably been quite an exciting experience for him. I located his phone, something I hadn't even been sure he could use, unplugged it and took it with me.

Since I knew that it was still possible that someone dishonest, or unobservant, enough might sell him a car, I had to take action to protect my dad, and the population, against that possibility. That was the day I went to the bank and made sure he could no longer access large amounts of money by placing most of it in another account I opened. Shaken, I drove home, still marveling at his audacity and cognitive chutzpah. He must have really pulled his scattered brain cells together to pull this off – which indicated to me how important it was to him.

I had certainly expected to deal with some unexpected events and behaviors – that's what dementia means, after all, but this one caught me off guard. Even understanding the importance of driving, I had underestimated his desire to hold on to something that had meant so much to him. Although what he did made me angry and afraid, it reminded me how devastating this disease had been for him, and that I needed to maintain my patience and compassion.

I also realized that I had truly become my own Father's parent: lecturing, taking away his phone, forbidding him to leave his room, and blocking access to money – as if he was a seventy year old teenager. It was a role switch neither of us would ever have wanted - the reality of role switching, in general, continued to sneak up on me as we continued our journey together.

*

All caregivers have a story about their loved one, dementia, and driving. All of us, at one point or another, have had to plot how to pry the car keys out of a loved one's hand; watch that loved one crash their car - or worse; or sneakily disable a car engine to prevent its use. It is one of the hardest parts about being a caregiver for someone with dementia. Since the day we are handed a license, driving represents independence, autonomy, and self-esteem. It is not surprising that our loved ones fight so hard not to give it up.

My mother's mother loved her sporty little car and, after so many years of letting my grandfather drive she enjoyed the independence of getting herself around after she was widowed. After my mom died, and as my grandmother got older, she still maintained that she only used her car to get to the store and back a few times a week and that she knew the way so well she could do it blind. (Which was good because she developed cataracts and began, literally, driving by brail – navigating the roads by using the protruding lane markers.) Finally, the community police put their foot down after too many traffic stops and my grandmother's (slightly battered) car was sold.

This is a topic that is on top of everyone's list of questions and concerns – everyone wants to know when, and how, to address the topic of driving. One of the most difficult tasks when assuming the role of authority has to be trying to stop a parent from driving. Caregivers swap ideas on this problem all the time, from secretly disabling cars, to stealing keys, to having doctors or licensing officials be the bad guys. There are a lot of possible answers and solutions but, as with many things, it depends on each individual family and situation.

I see stories on-line all the time about care receivers refusing to give up driving, and in a moment of confusion, causing a serious accident and injury to others. It is akin to allowing a drunk driver to get behind the wheel. Some dementia sufferers have serious accidents before their driving privileges are taken away. I am so grateful that Dad never had this happen, nor did he have an accident involving another person, which also happens.

There is a chance of being held legally liable for these accidents if it becomes known that caregivers allowed driving knowing the person was impaired. I know I would have felt guilty for the rest of my life if something like this happened. People's lives changed forever out of stubbornness and fear. Refusing to accept painful truths may comfort all of us briefly, but in the end it will cause more problems than it solves.

There is no perfect time, or way, to ask an adult to hand over their keys. When it becomes an issue of safety for *everybody,* however, it must be done. I think a good rule of thumb as to *when* it is time to take the keys is when you would no longer trust a child – yours or someone else's – to ride in the car with the impaired driver. Some people rely on the DOL to catch older drivers when they renew their licenses. Some ask their doctors to be the bad guys and explain the situation. Some people get rid of the car, or park it out of sight, or hide the keys, or remove the battery or some other vital piece of machinery.

Whatever works is what must be done. Everyone involved will have to do things they've never done, whether it's dealing with the emotions of taking control or dealing with the emotions around relinquishing it. Fortunately, there are more suggestions and solutions as the problem of dementia grows, but the issue will never truly go away because of what driving represents to all of us.

*

Problems caused by waiting too long to step into a possible dementia situation aren't limited just to driving. It is important to know all of the possible effects of waiting too long to step in and take over a loved one's affairs - effects that can have repercussions for everyone involved. Regardless of how the situation evolves, hesitating too long to take action can be detrimental to everyone. A problem becomes a crisis when it interferes with the safety and well-being of everyone involved. Things like mental and physical health, and financial stability can all be adversely affected by a delay in care or attention.

Where physical health is concerned, lack of action actively impedes diagnosis and medical intervention and increases the risk of dysfunction and injury. It can prevent an individual, or family, from seeking help and a diagnosis, which can prevent them from getting access to drugs that might help or slow the progression or an illness if taken early. There are certain dementia medications, for example, that lose their effectiveness as dementia progresses. A delay in diagnosis can cost a sufferer whatever assistance the drug would have provided.

Some dementia symptoms can be caused by disorders like strokes, hydrocephalitis, and malnutrition which are actually reversible so that damage to the brain and other systems can be prevented or ameliorated. Finding out whether these illnesses are what is causing cognitive problems is important before they get worse. Diabetes, malnutrition, and heart disease can all cause their own serious problems if undiagnosed – problems that might not have happened with medical care.

My particular situation with Dad happened slowly at first, then devolved quite rapidly into a crisis situation – being picked up by the police - which probably wouldn't have happened if I hadn't been so hesitant to take action. Dad exhibited signs of dementia several years before things hit critical mass. When we stepped in, his self-care and nutrition was very poor. I doubt he was getting very many nutrients at all since he was eating mostly carbohydrates, and he was fairly dehydrated. Poor nutrition and dehydration can contribute to and accelerate cognitive decline; if I had stepped in earlier, made sure he was eating and drinking properly and staying clean, he could have retained cognitive abilities longer.

Although we started him on Aricept when we received his diagnosis, the drug probably would have benefitted him more if taken earlier. The anti-depressants we put him on might also have helped earlier. Looking back now, I wish I had been willing to talk to him about his symptoms a little bit sooner.

*

In practical terms, a denial delay can also cost someone professionally and financially. Early stage and early-onset dementia can be misidentified or misinterpreted by employers and co-workers as laziness, poor performance, and inappropriate behavior. Misinterpreting these symptoms can lead to poor job reviews and even termination, when the individual should actually be on Disability insurance or a medical retirement, leading to a loss in income and/or respect and reputation.

All my life, Dad maintained a cone of silence around money, not even informing my mother how much his salary was or what their bank balance was. He lectured us repeatedly about the value of money, the value of being independent and of earning your own way. He could be shaming about money – forcing us to beg for our allowances and reprimanding us if we spent poorly or were financially unorganized. Yet when I stepped into his house to begin the process of arranging his life, his financial and business affairs were in shambles. I knew it was all a result of the illness affecting his judgment and abilities but I couldn't help but be angry after his constant lectures and expectations about precision around money and keeping good records.

Even with the dementia, money was one of the main things Dad's brain fixated on as the thing to remember and worry about. Whether that was because he was constantly concerned about it or because he historically equated it with control or independence was unclear. Ironically, if we had been a family able to discuss financial and legal arrangements and talk openly and honestly about money, and had done so early on, we may have been able to save him a lot of what he prized so highly.

It was difficult at first to determine what resources I might have available to me for his care. It was unclear how much money he had, or even whether he had any at all. To look at his living conditions, however, and the state of the house, was to conclude that he didn't have much. I assumed that Dad's salary had been fairly sizeable at the time of his retirement. I also knew that Boeing had offered him some sort of lump sum retirement deal, about which, of course, I had no details. He also had a pension through them that appeared to be in complete disarray. My parents had owned two apartment buildings that he sold after retiring. While I didn't know their worth, I assumed he had invested or saved whatever proceeds he had made.

My first task with his affairs was to embark on a little forensic accounting. I knew there had to be some money somewhere, but he repeatedly said that he was just living off small, quarterly dividend checks. It turned out that he was living off his dividend checks because he had lost track of his money, not because he didn't have any– ironically, he was worth over a million dollars.

When he finally allowed us to go through his papers and take a look at things, we found that he had become an accomplished amateur investor, taking the lump sums of money from his real estate sales and retirement, and investing them quite skillfully. Problems started, however, when the cognitive issues interfered with his maintenance of the funds and they were left to do the best they could. He also had portfolios in every investment firm I had ever heard of, and several I hadn't. It took me the better part of a year to complete the Sisyphean task of locating, contacting, and eventually consolidating them all.

The financial planner we eventually hired told us that Dad's portfolio had probably lost half of its value in the stock market problems of 2000, a loss which could have been avoided had he asked us for help in managing it. He had also lost a lot of money in duplicate fees by having accounts in so many different investment firms. We would end up spending a great deal of what he had accumulated on his care and housing, which might not have been the case if we had been able to talk about what was happening. Dad was so physically healthy that he could have obtained long-term care insurance when he was still relatively lucid which would have paid for much of the extensive care he would end up receiving.

*

Having a discussion about money is one of the most polarizing and divisive issues a family can face – family members often report it as the most difficult conversation to initiate, next to talking about the illness itself. Most families have at least a few issues around money, and many have severe ones. Family dynamics can be difficult and emotional enough; money adds an extra element to the mix. The perception of money as parental love, for instance, can unearth old jealousies and childhood hurts, as well as feelings of scarcity and resentment. The existence, or non-existence, of money can tear a family apart, when it comes to issues of inheritance, expectations, who will provide care and housing, and who is doing more, or less.

Parents may not want to divulge their financial arrangements, or lack thereof, out of privacy, independence, or even shame, and may deflect questions or discussion about it. It can also be hard for parents to see their children as competent grownups capable of handling decisions about money and other issues. If left unmonitored, finances can become disorganized and money can be lost to bad choices, bad investments, and ever-present scams.

I walked into Dad's apartment one morning to find several items I had never seen before: a printer, in its box; a new laptop, in its box; and two new digital cameras. When I questioned Dad as to where he had obtained these items, he happily disclosed the existence of a wonderful channel on television where you see something they are selling, you call in and tell them you want it, and they send it to you! Unbeknownst to me, he had opened up a credit line with QVC, or its equivalent, and had shopped till he dropped. I found the paperwork, called the company, and closed out his account, and sent back the items. If you'd asked me whether he was cognitively capable of these financial maneuverings, I would have said no, but I would have been proven wrong, so after that, I kept a closer eye on what he had, who he was calling, and what he was doing.

We all are starting to hear stories about scams that target the elderly and those with dementia. People who either call or show up at the front door with the intention of taking as much as possible from those who can't defend themselves. I hear many stories of care receivers losing checkbooks and cash, emptying bank accounts, giving money away, and losing money in bad investments.

Some adult children may put off a money discussion because they don't want to face a confrontation or bad feelings from their parents. Some just don't want to face the aging or eventual death of their parents, or find it too depressing, so they avoid discussions about financial and living wills, life insurance, and other arrangements.

In most families different people will have a difference of opinion where money is concerned, which means clear and honest communication is essential. It can be even more difficult when there is more than one family member involved, or trying to be involved, in the organization and decision-making. This can be detrimental when it comes to the question of housing and care, and how they will be paid for. Professional, twenty-four hour in-home care can be very expensive, and facility care costs even more.

Good financial arrangements can mean the difference between having one's pick of care options and facilities, or depending on Medicaid to pay for a cheaper facility, and can create crises and suffering or ease and comfort for all involved. The costs for caring and housing for an individual who is aging or has dementia are prohibitive. Care provided in the home by family members is the least expensive option, but costs for doctors, medication, necessities, and occasional professional aides can still add up.

Medicare does not cover any long-term care costs, unless it is skilled nursing care at a nursing facility and the patient continues to make progress in healing. Dementia does not count as a covered affliction by Medicare. Medicaid will cover facility care, but only at a designated rate determined individually, and only at certain facilities. In addition, someone applying for Medicaid must first spend virtually everything they have on care before they are accepted by the program.

*

Discussing these issues beforehand can help so much – indeed, would have helped us a great deal. Surely it is worth a little discomfort and difficulty. In addition, consider your own situation and whether your finances are up to the challenge of long-term care for yourself when the time comes.

Money, healthcare, driving, living alone, control – these are all part of the difficult terrain that we must navigate as caregivers trying to help our loved ones with change. There is no map, to point us in the right direction, no time table to tell us exactly when something needs to be done or an uncomfortable topic needs to be raised. We just have to start down the road and hope we don't hit anything along the way; or if we do, we have to hope it won't be fatal. The point is to get started, because procrastinating can cause more harm than good.

A Few Things I Figured Out.

- Colluding with the denial and not taking action could be detrimental to the physical and mental health of everyone involved: financial affairs could worsen; a delay in administering vital medication or medical care could result in more physical problems; it usually takes time to arrange essential legal, financial, and other matters, causing stress to everyone.

- It can be hard for the aging or ill to give up control and independence around issues like money and driving. Be patient and try to keep the lines of communication open. Remember, though, that it is now your job to keep them safe and well-cared for, which means making difficult choices and being seen as the bad guy. For good ways to keep loved ones from driving, check online forums, blogs, and Facebook pages, which are all great resources. If possible, have a trusted authority figure like a doctor, lawyer, or policeman take the driver's license. Secretly disabling a vehicle is also a viable option, as is "taking it to the shop to be fixed."

- Talk about financial arrangements, long-term care, Life insurance, and funeral plans early and often. Having good financial resources can mean the difference between many care and housing choices and poor-to-no- care and housing choices. Discuss inheritance issues with the entire family and determine beforehand who wants what and who will inherit what. Research long-term care insurance, savings and investment accounts, retirement accounts, and wills and trusts.

- Keep an eye on your care receiver's finances, as much as possible. Make sure they haven't opened up multiple credit accounts, or new checking accounts, and aren't ordering things over the phone or the television. Try to monitor who they hire to help do house repairs or other services, or tell them you will manage it for them. Scammers target the elderly all the time; quickly and quietly taking as much money as possible, and even threatening their marks with injury. As much as possible, keep an eye on the checking account, even holding on to the checkbook or offering to balance it for them and pay bills.

- Delays can cause serious medical issues. If we had stepped in for Dad earlier, some of the cognitive degeneration may have been stopped or at least slowed. Poor nutrition, dehydration, and poor self-care contributed to a rapid decline in his brain that we might have been able to help with. He did start taking Aricept, but it is a drug that is best taken in the early stages of dementia, and I think he probably started it too late – it didn't end up having much of an effect.

10.

The End of the Affair.

"Never regret. If it's good, it's wonderful. If it's bad, it's experience." Victoria Holt

Part of my story about becoming Dad's caregiver was the fact that my first romantic date in years occurred the same week as my planned move-in with Dad. The fact that my date, Charlie, and I got along and that I really liked him seemed like a gift from heaven as I was entering into one of the most difficult situations of my life. It seemed like Charlie and I had a lot in common, he made me laugh and think, we liked a lot of the same weird things and jokes, and I found him very attractive.

Our relationship choices are often affected by the circumstances of our lives at the time we make them. Sometimes we make poor, hurried, or uninformed choices because we are under stress or in a traumatic situation. We also make relationship choices according to the emotional patterns and expectations that have been laid down in us since childhood. Usually the kind of parents we had have something to do with it, as well. All of these things influenced my choice to latch on to Charlie so quickly.

I did not have a healthy relationship example in my parents, nor a good idea of what true nurturing looks like. My parents appeared to love each other but didn't appear to communicate about vital issues or feelings. Looking back now, I can see that they were living separate lives within their marriage, without much apparent emotional honesty. My mom's death devastated my dad, but as far as

I could see they had never truly been connected within their relationship.

I had been married before. I had gotten married in 1994 to my first husband for a lot of different reasons, if I am being honest; primarily because I didn't want to be alone, I wanted someone to take care of me, and, after several years of illness, I wanted to live a normal life. Because I didn't know how to find a real relationship, I chose a man who was emotionally immature, who probably got married for a lot of the same reasons I did.

We didn't know how to connect with each other or be emotionally honest together in relationship. We didn't know how to communicate clearly and really had no idea what marriage meant. When I started to grow and want more out of my life, and our relationship, he was unable to grow along with me and we separated. We were divorced a year later.

Charlie and I embarked on a serious relationship in 2004 – the first I'd been in since divorcing my first husband in 2000, and I thought I had dealt with a lot of the internal factors that caused me to make poor choices in men. When I met him, I thought that I had moved past some of my old patterns and mate picking mechanisms and could see him clearly. Turns out, I hadn't factored in what the extreme stress of moving in with my dad would do to my vision.

I thought I knew what a good relationship was *supposed* to look like. In a good relationship, there should be mutual communication; a mate should really be able to listen to you, and should really want to understand your issues. A mate should be trying to lift you up and should be interested in your continued growth. A mate should also put your well-being first, and consider you in all aspects of their lives. Ideally, you are doing these things in return.

In retrospect, my motivations were similar to those in my early twenties: I didn't want to be alone and I wanted someone to care for me. I kept picking mates through the lens of codependency: I'll care for you so you'll care for me. I needed help, Charlie seemed to fill the bill. He became a much-needed distraction from what else was happening around me. I jumped into the relationship far too quickly and started spending all the time I wasn't spending with Dad with Charlie.

What better way to mask the almost un-faceable facts of my father's illness and my residence in his falling-down house, caring for him, then a passionate, whirlwind, infatuated love affair? A love affair where I projected all my fear and grief and desire for someone to care for me (i.e. a Father) onto someone who clearly couldn't manage those projections for very long. (I guess it's no surprise that it didn't work out, although I wish I could have seen it earlier!)

Looking back now, I can see all of these projections and evasions of reality so clearly that they make me cringe a little. Losing a parent you love but with whom you shared a troubled relationship to something like dementia, and being forced to participate intimately in that process can be a little blinding, I guess.

I can see now that Charlie, while being the perfect escape vehicle, was not a stable craft. He was not the most emotionally-healthy person ever and there were many small red flags signifying his narcissism, depression, and other mental issues which I disregarded.

I really should have paid attention to statements like, "I really need to be the one in charge in a relationship." And, "If you aren't on my side, you're against me." And the classic, "I hate my job and I really want to just be a musician/rock star." But I was embarking on the toughest, most emotionally confusing thing I'd ever done. We started building a life together. And to his credit, Charlie helped me a great deal with Dad. In January of 2005, I gave up my studio apartment and moved in with Charlie, while still living with my father part of the week.

Charlie helped me agonize over every decision about Dad. When we chose an Assisted Living Facility for my father and moved him in, Charlie was there to move furniture and boxes, and help me weather my guilt over my dad's anger and grief. When the time came to clean out the family house and deal with forty years of hoarded furniture, junk and memories, he came with me every week of the six months it took us, keeping my spirits up and lending a valuable hand.

I believe that without Charlie, I would have had a much harder time getting through those first years of learning how to care for Dad, dealing with the detritus of his life, and experiencing the stress of watching him succumb to a terrible disease. For better or for worse, Charlie was part of the story and he played a very important part. I give him credit for the ways in which he showed up for me, and for how hard he worked to help me get through what was a very traumatic few years.

When it began, of course, our relationship had been based on real emotions and similarities, but it had, of course, also started during a time of great stress, drama and new feelings, a beginning that does not always lend itself to long-term stability. I began to see that Charlie's mental and emotional health had degraded over the years of our relationship, and he was exhibiting behaviors and attitudes that resembled those of a serious personality disorder.

These were things I had always been able to explain away or find other ways to deal with to defuse a situation. It appeared I had picked a man more closely resembling my father and his mental illness than I realized. I had hoped, as always, to find someone that would care for me, but again, as always, I was doing all of the caring – physically and financially.

This man did not want to help me grow, he wanted to keep me down in the depressed mud where he was. My happiness was not uppermost in his mind, which is what I have come to believe is of paramount importance in a relationship. Just like my father, he was selfish and did what he wanted, without concern for anyone else. He was happy to inflict his anger and misery on me no matter what effect it had on me.

I was supporting him while he followed his dream of being a musician (I know, I know), and he just couldn't seem to make it work, largely because he could be such an asshole. He insisted that everything be his way and nobody wanted to work with him. Even when he found a band that he liked, he found something wrong with them or some reason to quit.

I think what he really wanted was for the fame and success to be handed to him just because he thought himself so fabulous – grandiose behavior that signals narcissism, although I didn't realize it at first. The flip side of that coin was his fear that if he did put himself out there, it might turn out that he *wasn't* the rock god he fancied himself to be. It was easier to stay in the basement, practicing, and complaining about how unreasonable everybody else was.

In fact, this had become the territory of our relationship; him hiding out in the basement, either working on his computer or playing music, and me upstairs reading, working on my quilts, and writing. It was being borne in on me that this was not the healthiest of situations. The times we were together, we were arguing bitterly about his view of the world versus mine, and how much of a victim he was.

He was becoming much more volatile and violent, at times seeming to be outside of reality in his beliefs and demands, and the slightest thing could set him off. As in my childhood, I was never sure what I was going to get from a loved one. I began to walk, once more, on eggshells, which is what I later found out is a way of life for people living with someone who has Borderline Personality Disorder.

I was spending a lot of time unhappy, and he had become a person that I was no longer sure I wanted in my life. I had no experience with abusive relationships but I was becoming a little concerned for my safety, especially if I were to break up with him. It was so hard to decide what to do.

I was afraid of the immense physical effort it would take to cut him out of my life, and yet I knew I didn't want to live in this situation much longer. I was also afraid I would never meet anyone else and wind up old and alone. It is so hard when love dies and I couldn't seem to admit to it.

One afternoon in July, we were in the kitchen, arguing yet again. He had just finished one of his tirades about how bad it all was, and how I wasn't there for him, and that it just wasn't working out. His last words were to question whether we should stay together, saying that maybe we should break up - something he had said many times before, and which I had always protested against. I was leaning against the counter, and a sudden image filled my head. It was of a thick rope, snaking past me through the wall, and it was such a strong vision that I could almost touch the rope and feel the roughness of it against my hands.

At the same time, a voice in my head said that this was my lifeline and that if I didn't grab it now, it could be years before I got the chance again to get away. I hesitated for a second, then grabbed the rope in my mind. I told him I agreed with him that it wasn't working out and that we should definitely break up. We were both done in the relationship and it was time to stop making each other miserable. The shock on his face was, almost, comical.

Leaving the kitchen, I picked up my purse, phone, and car keys and walked out to my car. On the drive to Seattle I called a friend who arranged for us to meet downtown for lunch. She brought along another friend, and the three of us sat at a table while I described what had just happened and questioned whether I had done the right thing.

Both are in adult, healthy relationships and they explained to me exactly what I was missing out on and what a caring relationship is supposed to look like, i.e. someone who cares for you, wants the best for you, and is interested in helping you grow. Hearing this stated so plainly helped a lot. I knew that I had made the right decision. In fact, it felt as if I had already done all my grieving in the months leading up to the present moment and I felt our connection snap apart in that instant. I knew all of my feelings for him were gone; now I just had to weather the storms while I pulled him out of my life like a reluctant root. And it was a most difficult break-up.

A few years before, we had refinanced his house, so we were now co-owners. I didn't really want to keep the house, but the property market was bad and I didn't think we'd have much luck selling it, plus I was the only one who could pay the mortgage, since he had no job and no money, so it looked like I would have to buy him out of the house. This was irritating, largely because I had been paying the mortgage most of the time, anyway.

At first he refused to leave, trying repeatedly to change my mind or convince me that things could be different. I was exhausted from dealing with my chronic illness, and caring for Dad, and fighting with Charlie – fighting for my life, essentially. When he realized I was absolutely serious, he moved into the finished basement of our house while looking for a job and an apartment. It was not the best solution since I didn't really want to be near him and he could watch every move I made, but we finally agreed that he would be out by the end of October.

I was a little concerned that he might become enraged or hurt me, and it seemed like all I heard on the news were stories about women being killed by ex-boyfriends. It seemed like a particularly bad summer for that. Fortunately, nothing like that ended up happening. I did end up buying him out, he finally moved out and I was free, and relieved it was over. And I was, blessedly, alone.

I never cease to be amazed at the ways life can be surprising; what it takes away and what it may give in return. I had considered meeting Charlie a gift from the Universe to reward me for my selflessness. I don't regret the relationship, but it definitely turned out to be less of a reward than a booby prize. Perhaps I would have made different choices without the pressure of my father's illness.

The twists and turns my life has taken, especially when I thought all was settled or never going to change, have confused me, depressed me, humbled me and amazed me. It was incredibly difficult changing my life so drastically, and I feared that I might never meet anyone again. I am so glad I did, however, since making such a drastic change led me to even better events and people in my life.

A Few Things I Figured Out.

- Don't make important life choices when embarking on a challenging or difficult time in your life. You may not make the best decisions. It is okay to be alone during tough times, as well. Having a partner does make some things easier but don't accelerate a relationship because it is convenient.

- I would say to anyone in a similar situation: don't be afraid to leave an arrangement that isn't feeding and supporting you – don't stay with someone because you are tired, scared, or think you don't deserve better. Everyone deserves someone that wants to help them grow, not someone that keeps them squashed down. Although it took a lot out of me to finally end our bond and deal with the legal and financial issues, it was definitely worth the energy expended and the grief experienced to get out of a bad relationship.

- My experiences and beliefs might not mirror everyone's, but if there is one thing I have learned, it is that, if you're open to it, if you give yourself the chance and the space, growth can come out of even the most unlikely, difficult, or horrifying situation. Don't be afraid to trust in something new, don't be *too* afraid of change. Even if the only thing you can decide is what you <u>don't</u> want in your life, that can help guide you. Even though it was hard and painful at times I did get many benefits from our time together. I learned a lot about myself throughout our relationship and during our break up.

11.

Generations X, Y - and Y Me?

"In increments both measurable and not, our childhood is stolen from us – not always in one momentous event but often in a series of small robberies, which add up to the same loss." John Irving

When the average person thinks about caregivers – *if* the average person thinks about caregivers –– they usually think about someone in their late fifties to early seventies. They don't typically envision someone who's twenty to forty. This was, and is, of great interest to me since I am still one of the youngest caregivers I know. I was thirty-three when my father's shit hit the fan and I didn't have a clue about how to give care. I'd been running my own life for years, of course, but being responsible for someone else's? It felt far too soon to have to think about, and I felt far too young to have to do it.

I am not, however, unaccustomed to this phenomenon. I have always been ahead of the (age) curve, so to speak. My whole life I've had people tell me I was "too young!" for what was happening to me. I was "so young!" to lose a mother to cancer and was the only person my age I knew who had lost a parent, so I had no peers with which to share the many difficulties and challenges, and nobody to answer my questions.

I was "too young!" to have arthritis, becoming ill with rheumatoid arthritis when I was twenty-one, and therefore the only person in my peer group meeting doctors, discussing treatments and medications, and caring for myself. I joined the Arthritis Foundation-sponsored aqua aerobics class at the local pool and was the youngest person in the water by thirty years or more, surrounded by white hair and dentures, although they were all lovely, fun people.

I was "so young!" to be a caregiver, and found myself reading about caregivers who were in their sixties, or listening in a support group to people who were caring for parents and spouses who are in their eighties. (Of course, now is when I'd like people to tell me how young I am but at 43 I'm not hearing it anymore!) The thing is, I have rarely felt "so young!" I have always felt old. Due to events and circumstances beyond my control I have had to grow up fast; have had to tackle responsibilities way outside my skill set; and had to learn to deal with things far before my peer group. Much of the burden has rested on my shoulders. I've wanted to tell all of these people saying I was too young that I never *wanted* to deal with these things so young, they just happened.

*

Many psychologists divide life into four psychological stages designed to define an individual's identity. *Childhood* is characterized by the ego's dependency on the parents' world. In *First Adulthood*, from puberty to age 35, give or take, the dependency of childhood and reliance on the parent's help and regard is still a factor in the process of growing and adapting to the roles and rules of adulthood.

Second Adulthood marks the dissolution of dependency, the acceptance of responsibility, and the opportunity to become a singular individual, beyond the determinism of parents and cultural conditioning. The fourth stage, *Seniorhood,* involves mortality, which includes assessing one's life and achievements, and learning how to live with the realities of end-of-life.

Most people would accept this framework, to varying degrees, as a good, basic description of the stages of life. Theoretically, the experiences, events, skills learned, and relationships formed in each stage prepare an individual for the next. There are certain rites of passage that happen at certain ages, in a certain order - like driving, first love and dating, voting, living on one's own getting a job, marriage, and child-bearing. We are presumably equipped, knowledgeable, and ready for each stage of life.

Since we are accustomed to life events happening in a certain progression, at certain times in our lives, we presumably have the skills, abilities, and emotional maturity to deal with each one. When we are in elementary school, for example, we worry about how hard college is going to be, not realizing that by the time we have gone through the logical progression of grades and schools, we will be physically and mentally ready to be there.

As a society, we are geared towards this natural cycle - youth, adulthood, mid-life and parenting, later life and caring for elderly parents, aging and dying – it has always gone this way and we expect it to continue to go this way. There have always been exceptions to the natural order, of course, whether it involves the early death of a parent, an early-onset of illness, caring for children at a young age, or having to care for family members prematurely. However, we have been confident that most events will occur in the order in which they always have, that we will be of an age and understanding to be able to assume each set of responsibilities as they come, chronologically. One of the benefits of this orderly progression is that we have our parents and grandparents to help and guide us, the other is that we have a peer group experiencing it with us. Difficulties arise when events start happening out of order; when one person is dealing with something alone or that their peer group is unfamiliar with, or when expectations and maturity levels don't necessarily match up.

In many ways, I feel as if I simultaneously inhabit all of these stages, as if I have been consistently out of step with what most people consider the "normal" progression of events and stages of life, especially from the age of twenty and on. I feel like an oddity almost - a freak - as if I have been, in many small ways, an adult all of my life. When I look back on my childhood, it feels like from the beginning I was mature and knowing: like I am looking through a maturity filter, sepia and steady. I know this cannot be true, know for a fact I was at various times, childish, goofy, unformed, insecure, immature, dishonest, and trusting.

I believe it is true, however, that even as a child I was well aware that a certain level of maturity and adult behavior was expected of me. I can't remember when I didn't have a still center where I went to think about things and make decisions about what I would and would not do and say. In my family I was the peace maker, the Cruise Director, the one that tried to make everything smooth and okay, who took care of everyone else. So in a way, I have always been a caregiver, caring for everyone's emotional well-being. It's actually not surprising that I had little problem becoming accustomed to some of the aspects of dementia caregiving. I always felt that, at bottom, I was on my own: that if the ship went down with all hands, it was up to me to get to a lifeboat and save myself – nobody else was going to do it. It is possible that this is just how I remember it now – faulty recollections faded by the years and colored by therapy and introspection – but it feels accurate.

Perhaps this is what can happen to people like me, people who lose a parent at a young age, or who take on a great deal of responsibility, or suffer some other similar life-altering event. We are often accustomed to being the adult, with the attendant responsibilities. (This can come in handy, I suppose, when we are called on to undertake the care and feeding of someone else since we are accustomed to being the adult in the room.) We have generally experienced all of the age-appropriate life skills and emotions - however, we have most likely experienced them out of order or in out of the ordinary ways and have had to scramble to find information, resources, or assistance to help us learn how.

We have peers, with which we share some age-appropriate events and transitions, but we will always have a different sort of experience than they do. We are deprived, to a certain extent, of the normal progression of life experiences, growth opportunities, and learn abilities that serve to prepare us for the growing transitions and roles of adulthood; including, ultimately, the care of a parent or spouse and our own decline and death.

I realize that my experiences are a bit extreme and that I represent only a small percentage of people who have had a similar life progression, however, the point I am trying to make holds true.

Whether one has ten important life events happen out of order, or only one, it can leave an individual struggling and unsupported through some tough challenges. We become out of step with our age and maturity group, and with the expected cultural and chronological expectations, and we must struggle to find support and information that is appropriate to the situation.

When bad things happen, of course, you step up and work with what you have as best you can, but you know that everything would be easier if you were better equipped and there were more people around you managing the same thing. Even with all of my experience of dealing with things above my level of emotional maturity, having to be a caregiver really threw me. I wasn't prepared for it.

*

One of the "normal" expectations of caregiving - the act of living with and physically, mentally, and financially caring for a family member or loved one - is that an individual most likely won't have to undertake it until they are in their fifties or sixties, at the earliest, and often much later. Media, medical information, and other caregiving resources are aimed at an older demographic, and peer and support groups are generally made up of older people.

This demographic is expected to have their own lives mostly sorted: career in train, finances in order, house bought, families in process, affairs organized, etc. It is anticipated that older adults will have enough skills and experience already to do the myriad tasks and duties required of a caregiver. Therefore, caregiving will not begin until the caregiver is of an age to deal with it. Which, as we know, is not the rule anymore.

As caregivers get younger and younger this is where they will find themselves. This place of inhabiting more than one stage of adulthood because they are being asked to assume tasks and responsibilities ahead of their age and emotional pay grade. I have read that by 2037, the odds in favor of an individual between the ages of thirty and fifty-four becoming a caregiver could increase by 88%. These are pretty scary odds, especially when one considers the lack of preparation or awareness our society has around the growing number of people needing, and giving, care.

Over the last thirty to forty years health and health care has become a double-edged sword in that diseases are being researched and cured, new drugs are being discovered, lives are being extended, and people are being helped which means we have an older, sometimes chronically-ill population. Our country has become inundated with long-term illness due to better medical technology, environmental factors, and differences in nutrition and hygiene.

We have seen a marked increase in all of the dementia syndromes; various other neurologic diseases like multiple sclerosis and Parkinson's; different types of cancers; and various auto-immune and other chronic illnesses. The downside of extended life is that people are living longer with these natural illnesses and infirmities, even when they might prefer not to, and they need caring for.

The increasing use of the Intensive Care Unit and life-sustaining machines to keep our aging alive past the time when there is any quality of life is a case in point. We depend on hospitals and doctors for long-term care and treatment more than in the past, and most people die in hospitals instead of at home. There are more choices in terms of housing and caring for the ill and aging, but they are often expensive and/or unsuitable, leading to difficult choices and sometimes unsafe living conditions. We are caring for our ill loved ones for much longer periods of time, sometimes while living with our own chronic illnesses or physical aging issues.

*

In terms of the appearance of younger and younger caregivers, there are many reasons for the demographic shifts in caregiver age. Our social structures have changed over the last seventy-five years. People are getting married and divorced more often, over a longer period of time; women are having children later in life; and people are changing careers, and finding vocations, more often and later into life. The growth of early on-set dementias, and the fact that the aging are living longer, make it much more likely that individuals will be caring for a spouse, parent or grandparent when they are in their twenties, thirties, or forties.

While on the surface, it might seem as if the act of giving care would not be age-related, that the emotions and experiences are the same regardless of the age of the caregiver or the loved one they are caring for, I maintain that it really does matter. Younger caregivers require different types of support in their new role as giver of care, because they are facing different issues and going through different challenges – the ones that are appropriate to their age group – than those in their sixties and seventies.

As a caregiver, you will be responsible to make healthcare choices for your care-taker. Unless they are unlucky, or me, most people in this age group haven't had much experience with the medical world; illness, medication, doctors, specialists, and healthcare facilities. Get ready for an instant education in the human body and how it can go wrong. We must learn quickly how to find doctors, ask the right questions, decide on tests and procedures, and how to pay for all of this – which means insurance, Medicare and Medicaid. I know thank God for Google, which, I might add, didn't exist when I was embarking on *my* caregiving journey!

In addition, you will now be making financial and legal choices for your care-taker. Things like long-term care insurance, investments, retirement funds, and Social Security; as well as simple bank accounts, bill paying, and housing choices. Let's not forget about wills, medical directives, and trust and estate planning. Let's face it, many thirty and forty-year-olds are in denial about these things in their *own* lives, let alone dealing with them for someone else. How many thirty year olds have their wills prepared and have thought about long-term care? Many of them have never even bought a house or opened up a retirement account!

Even if you haven't had quite the event-laden life that I've had, being a caregiver before the age of, say, sixty, is going to be a strange, unexpected, and challenging event. Many people would say that caregivers are the same no matter what the age or sex, but this is not the case at all, which I can definitely attest to. It's not easy being a young(ish) caregiver, and whether others' experiences are as drastic as mine or not, I feel for the ones who are coming after me. Because there *will* be many coming after me

We need to change how we look at family structures, aging, illness, caregiving, and caregivers, because caregivers are no longer just seventy year olds caring for aging spouses. Caregivers are only going to get younger and younger and there are real and unique challenges facing them. Luckily enough, the media have already given us our own demographic name – "The Sandwich Generation."

A Few Things I Figured Out.

- As younger caregivers, we may not all share the same family situations. Some may still have one parent, or they have both parents and are taking care of a grandparent; they may have several step-parents and a big family; they may have their own children, be partnered, or be single; they may be teen-aged, a few years younger than I was or a few years older. Regardless of the specific details, one constant remains - we have all been asked to step outside of the natural order of aging, exit our peer group, and accustom ourselves to loss and new duties much earlier than the norm. This is a difficult thing to manage and there will be challenges we aren't used to. Grieve the loss, especially, of your youth and the fact that new things are being required of you.
- Changes in family structures, medical technology, and the growth of early-onset disease, and chronic, fatal illnesses like diabetes, heart disease, and cancer mean that caregivers will be getting younger. We are enduring a sharp learning curve

in terms of learning new and necessary skills, and balancing the needs and demands of several generations simultaneously. We are often forced to make life, family and career compromises. This can't help but resonate through all aspects of our lives.

- It helps to have people that understand the challenges of being a young caregiver. If you can't find friends or colleagues that share your new responsibilities, try to find a support group or go on-line. Think about starting your own support group in your area; the big organizations like the Lewy body Dementia Association and the Alzheimer's Association can help with how to start a group, how to find participants, etc. Check the message boards at local coffee shops, libraries, doctor's offices for potential groups.

- Google, Google, Google! There are so many more resources out there now than there were in 2003. There are countless forums, support groups, and Facebook groups you can find and be a part of that will definitely have people your age. Don't worry, you may feel alone now, but the odds are with you; there will be a lot more caregivers your age in the near future! Only one of my peers is now a caregiver, and that's a pretty recent development; in the next few years there will be more.

12.

The Sandwich Generation – Is It Just Baloney?

"First we are children to our parents, then parents to our children, then parents to our parents, then children to our children." Milton Greenblatt

As I pointed out, we are different people in our young(ish) adulthood than we will be later on. We have fewer or different skillsets and we may still be developing our lives, relationships, jobs, and even attitudes. People in their twenties, thirties, and forties are juggling all of the age-appropriate events, achievements, and relationships they are supposed to be juggling. At any one moment, these people are: dating, getting married, already married, going to school, working, changing jobs, discovering their vocation, traveling, getting pregnant, having kids, adopting kids, raising kids, dealing with special needs kids, building a house, getting a divorce, moving, dealing with cancer or chronic illness, and any number of other serious activities.

According to psychologists, this is the time of growing and adapting to the roles and rules of adulthood; hopefully, the dissolution of dependency and the acceptance of responsibility; and the opportunity to become a singular individual. This is a time is for building a foundation, learning the skills to support, feed, and house yourself, exploring who you are, and determining where you want your life to go. And yet, suddenly you are faced with the full-time burdens of caregiving. Caring for another person means essentially taking on their life, and their well-being; it is a huge consumer of time and energy. The sheer volume and variety of tasks and responsibilities that a caregiver must learn how to do can be overwhelming. Now that personal, developing life must be fit in around the demands of caring – the equivalent of several full time jobs taking place at the same time. Congratulations! You are now part of the "Sandwich Generation." Or is that just a simplistic term for a much more complicated issue?

I was twenty-seven when I first started seeing ominous changes in my dad, and thirty-three when I became a caregiver. Not a single person in my sphere was, or had been, a caregiver – not friend, colleague, or acquaintance – with the exception of my aunt who was taking care of my grandmother. Unfortunately, she lived in Detroit and we weren't close so it never occurred to me to ask her for help or guidance. Friends were supportive of my struggle but had no personal experience with caring – most of their parents were still hale and hearty.

It was difficult for them to understand some of the issues I was facing and none of them had referrals or much advice they could give me. Once again I was way ahead of my age group. (It's funny to look at the situation now - my father will be long dead by the time my friends start having to care for their parents. I'll have to help my husband with my mother in law but after that I'll be done, watching everyone else go through it. I'll be a gold mine of information.)

I took on my dad's entire life, along with my own. Among other things, I was suddenly responsible for: financial decisions, bill-paying, investing and retirement accounts, and tax-paying; record-keeping, research, organizing social security and Medicare; making healthcare choices, organizing legal documents and funeral plans;

housing maintenance and insurance, housework and cooking, entertainment, and personal care.

I'm used to managing money, time, and people, I'm detail-oriented, and I'm good at decision making but when you're making important decisions for someone *else's* life, it becomes a whole new ballgame of angst and anxiety. Accustomed as I was to more mature responsibilities and expectations, I still really needed some guidance and support but I could not find one bit of information on how to manage an experience that, while common in later ages, was not in my demographic.

The few support groups that I found were filled with older people, who were at a vastly different stage in their lives. In addition, most of them were taking care of a spouse, not a parent, which can be a different experience altogether. As nice and supportive as they were, and they were, it wasn't the same as talking to someone my own age. I was on the receiving end of a lot of disbelief and pity from people when I explained what I was doing. (You're so young!) Apparently, even those people who are intimately acquainted with caregiving, either professionals or long-term family caregivers, don't envision thirty or forty year olds.

I always turn to books for information and support and I found a few books on the subject of caregiving, but they were all aimed towards people in their late fifties, sixties, and seventies. There were no books specifically aimed towards my demographic. Most of the books currently on the market were written by and for baby boomers; unfortunately, it's the baby boomers who are now becoming the patients/subjects. (It's worth noting that, at the time, there weren't that many great resources – book, internet, support group, organization – for a*ny* caregivers. I've noticed that it is only in the last six or seven years that there has been an explosion in caregiver support through the above outlets. Yay.)

The first book I found that resembled my situation was called, *The Family on Beartown Road.* It was about a woman my age who had moved her increasingly demented Father into their home and was caring for him, and writing about the experience. I devoured that book for hints and clues about what *I* was going through, as well. The biggest difference between us was that she had kids. She was part of a growing societal niche called "The Sandwich Generation." After reading the book, I started seeing that term popping up in a lot more places.

Sociologists and others who are interested in this sort of thing have recognized the growing trend of younger caregivers and assigned them a niche and a name, "Sandwich Generation." In other words, people in their thirties, forties, and fifties, who are still raising their children, but who are also caring for ill or aging parents. They are the filling "sandwiched" between two generations of individuals needing care.

Those of us who actually give care could probably also give a crap about having a name to call our group. We're too busy *doing* what it is the "Sandwich Generation" is supposed to be doing to care whether we have an official designation. However, the benefit to a catchy title is a growing awareness in the media and the minds of others about the special circumstances, burdens, and struggles that people in this demographic are facing. And those burdens and struggles can be overwhelming. Let's face it, at this age, most of us are planning on changing our *child's* diapers - not our *parents'*. Imagine the difficulty of raising a young family while at the same time trying to care for an aging or ill parent. These caregivers are caught in the middle of the, surprisingly similar yet mutually demanding, needs of two generations, forced to balance work, home life, and care in an increasingly unmanageable way.

This is where things got a little hard for me again, in terms of a peer group. Yes, the people belonging to the "Sandwich Generation" were the same age as me, but I don't have children, so I don't have the specific problems that they have of being caught in the middle of two generations needing care. I can certainly understand the problem, however, and I feel for them deeply, but it felt like, once again, there was no information specific to my situation. I didn't even start to see media about this group designation until a few years after I started caregiving.

There can be other groups of younger caregivers that don't quite fit into the "Sandwich Generation." For example, *really* young caregivers – kids from eleven to twenty who are caring for ill family members. This is a growing, and disturbing, reality: teenagers heroically giving up school, friends, and social lives to meet the needs of a mother, Father, grandparent, or sibling. They are making these sacrifices because there isn't sufficient money for professional care, and there isn't anyone else who can do the job. These young people need support, and some PR too, because this is a trend that, unfortunately, appears to be growing.

Another group that comes to mind are people taking care of *spouses* as well as, potentially, the children they share with that spouse. Again, with the upswing of early-onset Alzheimer's and other dementias, and growing instances of illnesses like certain kinds of cancer, heart disease, diabetes, and stroke, people may become ill at a relatively young age. The potential that wives will be caring for sick husbands, or husbands will be caring for sick wives – while at the same time caring for children – is growing.

This is again why I empathize with, and try to talk about, the people who don't quite fit in a group. Even though you may only have one burden "sandwiching" you in (and are therefore in more of an open-faced sandwich, as it were) you are still in a tough place. However, I think it might be fair to say that even if we don't have kids, or we are kids giving care, or we are caring for a spouse and kids, we *are* part of a *type* of sandwich generation, in that we are stuck between our own needs and lives and the needs of our care receiver.

*

The demands of giving care, usually to an aging or ill parent, can put a terrific strain on a young(ish) family. Emotions like resentment, anger, and grief may fester if not discussed honestly, openly, and often. Relationships can fray and split apart under the burdens of caregiving. Those individuals who already have a partner may find that the chores and responsibilities of caregiving can interfere with a relationship. Spouses may feel neglected or abandoned or as if they must carry the entire burden of the household while the caregiver deals with their care receiver.

Finances can become strained and living situations can become uncomfortable.

Non-married partners may feel that this exceeds what they signed up for as a boyfriend/girlfriend, and that the demands of the care receiver, and the stress of the caregiver, are too much. I met a male caregiver on-line who had moved his demented mother in with himself and his girlfriend, who sounded like a paragon of patience and kindness. When I asked whether his mother caused strain between them, he said that occasionally they felt the stress but that his girlfriend helped out a great deal with his mother's care and entertainment and rarely complained. I've seen marriages crack under the strain of caregiving so to see a relationship like this last was pretty impressive.

Caregiving burdens can be tough for those young(er) caregivers who are taking care of spouses. With the advent of multiple marriages some women in their late thirties and early forties are married to older men who are developing dementia in their late fifties and sixties. These women, and a few men, are having to give up and grieve the spousal relationship, while they are still fairly young! They are having to give up the years of love, communal life, and activities that both members of the couple had counted on having together.

Joanne Koenig Coste, who wrote the groundbreaking, *Learning to Speak Alzheimer's,* was in this situation. Her husband manifested dementia in his forties, while they still had very young children. In that moment, she lost the future they had envisioned together. At that time, in the seventies, there were almost no resources for caregivers. The Alzheimer's Foundation hadn't even been formed. She was forced to find ways to financially support the entire family, care for her husband's growing needs, care for her children, and have some sort of life for herself. That she was able to do it, and then come up with, and write about, an amazingly compassionate, commonsense technique for dealing with those suffering from dementia is a testament to her character.

Children can unfortunately be affected negatively by the demands of caregiving. The caregiver may lack the time, energy, or money that they formerly had for their children. Children may not understand new roles or limits, and they may resent new living arrangements and the demands of the care receiver. Children may also fear the manifestations of the care receiver's illness. The families that communicate early and often about what is happening and what is to come are the most successful in meeting everyone's needs.

Individuals who are giving care may put off having children because they don't have the time or energy and can't foresee when they will, or don't want to bring a new life into a potentially unstable situation. I was already considering not having children when my father became ill but knowing that I was responsible for his needs for years to come (ten and counting!) was enough to make me finalize my decision.

And, as my own experiences illustrate, those individuals who don't already have significant others may make poor choices when looking for one out of exhaustion, financial reasons, fear of being alone, a desire to be cared for, or a desire to escape. They may choose someone they secretly hope will care for them more than is healthy or normal, or unwittingly choose someone they have to care FOR. I can personally attest to the dangers of dating when caregiving.

When I decided to move in with my dad to be his caregiver, and started dating at the same time, I acted unwisely because I wasn't aware enough of what I was doing and why. It is impossible to be careful and discriminating - as one needs to be when choosing a mate – when one is going through the emotional upheaval of caring for one's father. I should have known that being unsure of how I would integrate the demands of my new duties with the demands of a new relationship, as well as unsure how I would even *explain* my new situation was a red flag. If I had to do it again, however, I would definitely not mix the two.

I decided the first person I dated (Charlie) was *the One,* and immediately dumped my fear, rage, and grief about my father into the relationship – the equivalent of putting one's fingers in one's ears so as not to hear what one doesn't want to hear. As it turned out, the relationship lasted for a while, but ultimately proved unhealthy and unsustainable. Admittedly, I probably would have been a much bigger mess emotionally during the first years of caring for Dad without the distraction of a relationship, so there was some benefit.

There is no question that getting involved with someone so seriously at the same time that I was dealing with the hugeness of my father's dementia was a mistake. I believe I would have chosen a healthier partner without the stress of caregiving influencing me. I ended up caring for *two* men who couldn't care for me back and couldn't appreciate the care I was giving them. I am sure my vision was clouded to those warning signs I saw at the very beginning because I was so desperate to have some kind of normal – young - life just when I was having to do something abnormal.

*

Taking on the duties of caregiving can also affect existing social networks and how one is perceived by one's "group". Friends, acquaintances, and even family members may have difficulties adjusting to the altered circumstances, new behaviors, and responsibilities of the caregiver, and they may not know how to react. I was talking about elder care, Powers of Attorney and assisted living facilities while my friends were working on their careers, traveling and starting families.

We become accustomed to, and invested in, the different positions we and our friends hold in each other's lives; when an individual must assume a new position, it causes ripple effects throughout the whole social network. Confused by new dynamics in relationships that have had traditional boundaries, individuals don't know how to respond or react. Unsure how to help or hesitant to interfere, friends stop calling. Overwhelmed by the demands of their new position, caregivers vanish from sight. Supportive bonds fray just when a caregiver may need them the most.

Professionally speaking, caregiving can take a serious toll on the life of younger caregivers. There is really no way for one's professional life not to be affected by the burdens of giving care. Working caregivers, many of whom are balancing demanding jobs with the needs of their care receiver, often have to put up with the perception by bosses and co-workers that they are slacking or not interested in advancement or lack the "killer instinct" the job requires. They may be passed up for promotion or for good projects because of a perception that they are not committed. One-third of caregivers decreased their working hours and almost 30% passed up a promotion or assignment because of caretaking. About one-fifth took a leave or switched to part-time, 16% quit altogether.

Caregivers may refuse promotions, important trainings, and even better jobs at different companies because of the demands of caregiving. Career advancement may be halted for the duration. Caregivers may put off a dream career due to lack of time or energy or be unable to pursue or complete undergraduate or advanced educational studies. Big decisions like a new house, living in a new area, graduate school, or travel will probably also be deeply affected by the demands of caregiving.

On the plus side, more companies are promoting working from home, thanks to the Internet, and flex time for childcare. The Family Leave Act is at least one step towards better support of our caregivers. Younger caregivers should make sure that their employers are fully aware of the care situation so that a better work environment, hours, and salary can be worked out.

There is a gender bias in caregiving, as well. Caregiving is still perceived as more of a feminine chore, requiring special nurturing and compassionate skills that women are purported to possess more than men, who are expected to be in the corporate world, professionally earning. More than 80% of unpaid caregivers are women and yet many of these women hold down full time jobs, while caring for and raising their own families. Women must make impossible choices between their professional job and their unpaid ones, often exhausting themselves and/or giving up work hours and income to meet the needs at home. Women curtailing work time has long-term consequences – lower wages, fewer benefits, and reduced retirement savings, since quitting a job means less eligibility for social security. They may be unable to contribute to retirement plans and since these are things best started in one's twenties and thirties, this will have a significant effect on future economic stability.

No matter what your age, when it comes to caregiving, something is always sacrificed, whether it's family time, personal time, job advancement, money, or dreams of a higher education. I'm not saying that, as younger people, we are incapable of taking these challenges on – far from it. I have spoken to others my age who are facing their unexpected duties with compassion, grace, and intelligence. One can still have a life and a family and be a caregiver but it is more difficult, especially when one's peer group is focused on different things and there is little understanding of, or support for, what one is going through.

*

When we are dealing with tough events, we want to know if other people similar to us in age and experience are going through the same challenges, and we want to know how they are doing it. We want to know we are not alone. As I'm writing this, I realize that I'm not really offering a cure or fix; after all, the caregiving must be performed regardless of our awareness that we are too young to be doing it. However, I still think that, while hearing about experiences or receiving support from an individual of *any* age is comforting and helpful, getting it from someone who is right where we are is vital. Given this, I'm advocating for wider awareness on *who* is having to give care. We must give everyone, regardless of age, the acknowledgement, support, and access to age-specific tools, information and resources that will help them succeed in these difficult tasks. The old sources of information and support will no longer be enough. If we can bring this growing reality – this changing paradigm – into the forefront of our discussion, then we can begin to change the type of information and support that is out there.

I think it is the tendency of generations like the Baby Boom and Generation X to be introspective and forthcoming with our thoughts and feelings that will help us get through. We might be considered to be more self-involved and self-centered than previous generations, however, we are also perhaps more resourceful in terms of seeking therapy, talking to friends about problems, or seeking out methods of self-initiation through books and workshops. We talk about personal matters, and we're likely to try self-help. Indeed, I read, and continued to read, any self-help book I could find about caregiving, self-care, and making more of one's life. I also had a dedicated therapist through the entire process.

It is hard to have had to take on these "adult" responsibilities so early. It is hard not having parental guidance and company. I miss my mother terribly every time I see a woman my age and her mother out walking or shopping, or need some advice about a difficult problem. I miss my father when my husband and I go to a car show or when I want to ask him something about finances or buying a house or car. Coming to terms with his illness and the need for me to be mature and take charge also made it clear that I no longer had the comforting bulwark between myself and my own mortality that parents often represent.

After a lot of research, a great deal of talking to other caregivers, and the benefit of hindsight, I can see even more clearly where some of the problems lie for younger caregivers and the kind of help and support that might come in useful. It was entirely due to the lack of information on my specific situation that I wrote my first book, so I could let all the younger caregivers that I knew must be out there that they weren't alone, and provide them with some age-specific information. This book is a way to elaborate further and help more people.

A Few Things I Figured Out.

- We need more preparation and support that is geared towards our needs, our lives, and the ways in which we handle problems. Fortunately, that information and help is becoming more readily available. Look for books, blogs, Facebook groups, support groups, and organizations to provide the help you need. I had to learn as I went along but there are more resources now, such as; classes on how be a caregiver given by local hospitals, classes on finances and investing, and information on wills, advanced directives, and other legal issues. Empower yourself with information. You should be thinking about all this stuff for yourself, anyway.

- The challenges of caregiving can put stress on all aspects of life – a life that is most likely still in the process of forming. Be aware of added stress to spouses and children. It is important for me to add, however, that any of these relationships can also be strengthened by a caregiving situation. Families may draw closer together and bond under the challenges. They may take on the difficulties together and help each other with care of the care receiver. If there is good communication, clear boundaries, healthy expectations, and love, many good things are possible.

- Decide carefully when making job changes, decisions about school, or even housing decisions – don't let caregiver stress push you into making the wrong decision. Be careful when dating; make sure you are looking at your potential mate clearly. Make sure employer are aware of the situation and restrictions so that a better job experience can be arranged. Most employers will be understanding. There are retirement options for those who aren't "officially" employed. Be aware of the issues around your future retirement. Act slowly and carefully in all situations. Good communication, good boundaries, and giving yourself time and space can help in almost any situation.

- Talk to a therapist, spiritual advisor, or trusted friend. Use your age and your willingness to share your feelings to your advantage and get help. It is a benefit that we are willing to share more, to be more open, and to discuss our issues and problems with the therapeutic community. We need better, cheaper access to that support, however. There are community resources that can help with sliding-scale therapy.

- There are, in fact, teenage caregivers – children giving up their childhood to care for an ill family member. Imagine if you were having to meet the challenges you are now meeting when you were a teen! A survey in 2005 by the National Alliance for Caregiving, reported that at least 1.3 million children ages 8 to 18 help care for a sick or disabled relative, with 72% caring for a parent or grandparent. Caregiving raises the risk for depression and anxiety in child caregivers. These young people are isolated and unable to bring home friends, they are usually lacking sleep, which makes for difficulties completing class work, and they are being asked to perform tasks that even adults would hesitate to do. They need our help to spread media awareness. Encourage younger caregivers to write books and/or blogs about their experiences; to join or form peer-appropriate support groups; to get help from school counselors or administrators.

13.

Who the Hell Is Lewy body?

"LBD is not a rare disease. It affects an estimated 1.3 million individuals and their families in the United States. Because LBD symptoms can closely resemble other more commonly known diseases like Alzheimer's and Parkinson's, it is currently widely underdiagnosed. Many doctors or other medical professionals still are not familiar with LBD." *What is Lewy body?* LBDA website, www.lbda.org.

Believe me when I say that I have been in all manner of healthcare-related buildings in my day. Doctor's offices, clinics, hospitals, surgical rooms, Assisted Living facilities, nursing homes, skilled nursing facilities – you name it, I've seen it; either because of *my* illness or my dad's. I can say with all honesty, however, that, pre-caregiving, I had never seen the inside of a Geriatric Psychiatric facility, nor did I ever expect to, or particularly want to.

Not that many people have, actually, because there aren't that many of these facilities and they perform a pretty specialized function – caring for the neurological needs of the geriatric population. In fact, we were lucky that they had a bed for my father when he needed one. Which is another thing I never expected, although I probably should have: the fact that my dad might end up in a Geri-Psych ward, yet here he was, inhabiting a small room in a locked ward with other aging patients.

After I moved Dad into the facility, it took at least six months before I didn't flinch every time the phone rang, convinced that they were calling me to come and get him. All seemed to be going well and I had fervently hoped that he would comfortably live out his days there. One afternoon, I got the call about an incident involving my father in the common room of his Facility. The call came from the Nursing Director at the facility, letting me know that they were waiting for the ambulance to take Dad to the hospital.

It was difficult to determine the order of events but from what I could decipher, Dad had objected to another resident petting the cat that lived in the dementia wing, a cat he considered his. He had threatened the resident, a man, but had not hurt him; instead he had picked up and thrown a chair, and when he was approached by caregivers, he threw a punch at one of them, although it hadn't connected with its target. I could hardly believe it. My self-controlled father, so pacifist that he wouldn't even let a letter opener into our house, was swinging for the fences with lounge furniture. It was almost incomprehensible. The nursing staff had called an ambulance and sedated him and were sending him off to the hospital – in essence, dumping the problem onto someone else.

The ER was a nightmare, Dad was disoriented and angry. We hadn't even had the chance to be there with him since they called us so long after the event. He had already been admitted by the time we arrived. I'm sure he was scared and confused. Many ERs will give calming or anti-psychotic medication to patients if they are agitated or acting out, and those meds are generally harmful for the elderly and people with dementia.

My dad spent several days in the hospital, drugged up to a certain extent, but still causing problems. Several times, he managed to pull himself together cognitively, what we call "showtime"- a phenomenon during which a dementia patient can make a huge effort to appear cognitively able and healthy for a few hours. He would argue with me and the doctors about what was going on and what he wanted to do. He didn't remember the incident at all. The Assisted Living facility refused to take him back until he had spent some time under observation, preferably at a Geriatric psychiatric ward. This actually made me really mad and made me feel like they were trying to avoid their responsibilities to him and to our family, although I also knew that they had a responsibility to their other patients and families.

It was difficult to find him a bed in a ward, since there were only three Geri-psych wards in our area, and I can only imagine the flurry of faxes and admitting papers that were flew back and forth as everyone argued about where he was going to go. Finally, somehow, we were able to get him admitted into a ward, where he stayed for several weeks, over-medicated and deeply unhappy. Until that moment, he had never taken anything stronger that Lexapro, an anti-depressant, and Aricept for his illness, and I hated how slow and drugged up the anti-psychotic medication made him. Fortunately, his friend and aide, Del, was willing to spend most of each day with him – feeding, dressing, shaving him, and just keeping him company.

I visited as often as I could, and it never got easier seeing Dad there, sitting dumbly at a table, dressed up in layers for warmth, as other seniors sat, immobile, next to him or drifted ghost-like down the hallway. The only good moments were sitting with my father during lunch time, watching as he devoured his cup of chocolate ice cream – obviously still taking pleasure in the sweet, cold treat.

I went to the hospital to meet a social worker who would hopefully help me decide Dad's immediate future, walking down the squeaky-floored hallway lined with doors with signs on them saying, "Do not let patients out. Check the door has locked behind you!" On my visit, I struggled with several emotions; the most important being the fear that they would discharge Dad to the Assisted Living Facility who would turn around and kick him out, leaving me to care for him

Fortunately, the social worker had some ideas for me about when Dad could be moved and what medications to keep him on, and he kept in touch with the Assisted Living Facility about when my father could return. I'd been hopeful about him returning to what was his home, but I still wasn't sure they would take him, which made me a little angry because what were they doing there after all, but helping people who have dementia? They seemed a little too anxious about their own liability and a little too dismissive of Dad's needs.

I'd never heard of Alzheimer's disease making patients aggressive and combative (which just goes to show I hadn't done nearly enough reading!) If this was Alzheimer's, as we'd been told, how come no one had ever told us that something like this could happen? What were we going to do if it happened again? I had hoped that the disease would just continue to progress slowly and quietly as it had done all along, but I realized this was no longer likely.

After he moved back to his Assisted Living Facility, drugged up on Zyprexa, an anti-psychotic medication, I took him to his primary care physician, who read his charts carefully, examined Dad, and watched him walk. She was the first one who mentioned the possibility that he might have Lewy body dementia and not Alzheimer's. To which I said, "Who the hell is Lewy body and what does he have to do with my father?" Imagine my surprise to find out about different types of dementia, each with their own paths of progression, symptoms, and contraindications. We had just entered a new part of dementia country and I was lacking the right map.

*

At the beginning, during the diagnosis period of my father's process, nobody even mentioned to me that there was more than one type of dementia. Alzheimer's has the best PR of all of the dementia syndromes, and since there is no way to know for sure until a brain autopsy after death, it's usually the first guess of most doctors and was what all the medical personnel decided Dad suffered from.

I did the best I could with Dad, according to the excellent books, *How to Speak Alzheimer's,* and *The 36-Hour Day,* both very helpful. Some of the symptoms they described didn't quite match, either, especially since at first, Dad was pretty high-functioning. Even then, there were ways that it didn't seem to fit. He was relatively lucid and able in some ways but not in others, better on some days than others, but I figured Dad was just being his usual unique self. Eventually, it didn't really seem to matter – we were dealing with physical symptoms that resembled Alzheimer's so that was how I reacted.

Since most people also usually have a mix of dementias, starting with the most common one isn't such a bad thing. The reason it is important to get a correct diagnosis, however, is because there are differences between the dementias. Different dementias affect different portions of the brain, causing different symptoms and behaviors that can be surprising and even unsafe if they are unexpected. There are medications that are contraindicated for some dementias but not others and there are activities and medical procedures that should not be undertaken by people with certain dementias. There are also certain environmental factors that are more important to some dementia sufferers. This would turn out to be the cause of Dad's episode, although I didn't know it: "What the hell is this all about?" was my first reaction after Dad's melt-down. That and, "What now?"

My dad's doctor was very patient and kind. She told me that Lewy body (LBD) was a Parkinson's-related syndrome, and she gave me a quick list of symptoms and behaviors that seemed to fit the aggressive outbreak that had brought us to this place. She lessened the dosage of anti-psychotic medication that he was on and sent us on our way, back to the facility, with the warning that environment and atmosphere could be very important to a Lewy body sufferer, including excess noise, lights, people, and input.

Whereas Alzheimer's tends to begin in a specific part of the brain – the learning centers, causing problems with memory - it is impossible to guess in what part of the brain Lewy body dementia will blossom. Lewy bodies are abnormal proteins found in many different areas of the brain. They cause a depletion of the neurotransmitter dopamine, which causes Parkinson's symptoms, and acetylcholine, which disrupts perception and thinking. It becomes difficult to accurately predict what functions and systems will be affected.

The main differences we see in symptoms between Alzheimer's and LBD were the things that confused me the most about Dad. There may not be as much memory loss with LBD, and cognitive abilities, attention levels and alertness can change from day to day. This totally matched how Dad was able to manage in some ways but lacked abilities like cooking and caring for himself. He was definitely more aware than most of the people in the dementia wing with him, and that caused him a lot of grief. Those with LBD also suffer more often with visual hallucinations and delusions, and often have a sleep disorder that causes them to act out their dreams. This supports the vivid dreams that Dad had several times, after which he was sure that what had happened in the dream had actually taken place.

Dad never showed any symptoms resembling Parkinson's until the doctor watched him walk after the psychiatric episode and realized he was shuffling and couldn't pick up his feet. I didn't know that some individuals start out with the cognitive problems and eventually develop physical symptoms resembling those of Parkinson's, like shuffling, difficulty picking up feet, balance issues, rigid muscles, and tremors. Some people start out with the Parkinson's symptoms, and develop the cognitive issues later.

Lewy body sufferers can still possess many of their memory functions and memories: any part of the brain can be affected and can begin to malfunction and lose neural connections. The relationships between thinking and acting become cut off so that a thought no longer leads to its logical action. Cognition can actually improve and then worsen on a daily basis, which leads to caregiver confusion.

Lewy body sufferers can exhibit sleep disorders, including REM sleep behavior disorder and restless leg syndrome; disorders that may manifest years before cognitive issues. Lewy body may affect the autonomic nervous system, causing issues with blood pressure; the ability to regulate body temperature; bladder and bowel control issues, including nausea; dizziness; and sexual dysfunction. Lewy body can also cause depression and apathy.

The best metaphor I've heard to describe the effects of the disease is the following: imagine a patterned blanket that someone has thrown acid on, there are big and small holes, and there are also sections of whole blanket. Feeling along the blanket, you will encounter either holes or cloth, randomly and unpredictably. The pattern of the blanket as a whole has been distorted. This is what happens to the brain of a Lewy body patient.

Looking back on it now, and given my research, I think, "Of course! Of course Dad had Lewy body dementia. It all makes sense. All the crazy symptoms, and changes in lucidity and the different reactions and progression from Alzheimer's. This was what was going on!" It was actually kind of liberating, and validating, to know the truth given that I had always felt that something didn't fit. I had felt for years that there was more going on behind his eyes than he let on, more that he understood and remembered. A more defined diagnosis also helped explain what had made him go nuts and gave us strategies to hopefully avoid it happening again.

Some of the most significant differences with LBD, as well as other dementias like Frontotemporal Dementia and Vascular dementia, are behavioral. Whether it is believing in delusions of paranoia and acting accordingly; or seeing and hearing things that aren't there and interacting with them, sometimes benignly, sometimes dangerously; or just experiencing and acting on feelings of fear, anger, aggression, and anxiety – these dementia sufferers can prove difficult to handle. Unfortunately, the prejudice against those suffering from the more behaviorally-involved dementias is alive and well – in the one environment where it should be most accepted and welcome - dementia facilities.

There are stories everywhere about caregivers who are struggling to place their loved ones. About facilities that either wouldn't accept their loved one with LBD or asked them to leave because the facility wasn't equipped, or prepared, to deal with any dementia behavior out of the "ordinary." Every caregiver knows that ordinary is not a word one can apply to dementia. These poor individuals are forced to search for facilities that will accept their loved ones, sometimes settling for substandard care. When Dad got aggressive *one* time, his facility almost didn't accept him back. The stigma against "difficult" dementia patients is incredibly harmful.

Lewy body sufferers often take the brunt of this stigma due to the extreme symptoms of the disease – but Alzheimer's can cause some pretty strange and taxing behaviors as well. Facility directors are wrong in thinking that refusing Lewy body sufferers will keep things neat and tidy. I realize that many of these facilities are underfunded and understaffed, but where are else are dementia sufferers, regardless of their behaviors, supposed to go but dementia facilities?

It seems necessary that we somehow change the perceptions that facilities have of certain types of dementia so that we can improve the ability of the facility to take on every sufferer, not just the quiet ones. We could also pass laws to improve the pay and education that facility caregivers get so that they are better equipped to handle problems. Improved financial support of facilities by the government is also possible, so that they are able to accommodate all dementia sufferers. There ARE ways to deal with these types of dementias without constant fear, drugging, or confinement – it just comes down to proper education and support of facility staff.

As time went by, I began to consider that keeping Dad in the big facility was no longer the best thing for him. Although he didn't have another big episode, his behavior was definitely changing. I could see that the busy-ness and noise of the dementia wing was bothering him. He was also being watched and monitored closely by the staff in case of another outburst and I could actually see that this affected him. I could tell that he could feel the weight of their fear and expectations, which really made me angry. Was this not a dementia wing? Does dementia not sometimes include outbursts and unsocial behaviors? Were these caregivers not supposedly trained in how to deal with these behaviors? Apparently not.

After talking to the director and the dementia wing nurse, it seemed like everyone agreed that the facility was no longer the best place for Dad. It was time to move him, negating my hopes that he would spend the rest of his days in one place – a place he had been for years and was comfortable in. We needed a place that would accept Dad's behavior problems; something that might be a real sticking point. Lewy body, not widely understood and with difficult behaviors and symptoms, could make facilities leery of accepting someone who suffered from it. So, my best laid plans came to naught, and I was having to make new ones. Personally, I am not the best at accepting change, but as a caregiver for someone with dementia, you have to be flexible. My idea that he could live out his days in one place, while a good one, was no longer viable.

*

Luckily, I was referred to a woman who specialized in placing people with dementia. These specialists are paid a commission by whatever facility is chosen, however, the fee was set by the State to avoid fraud and was the same for every facility. It seemed like a really good system to me. I found it personally interesting that in just the few years since I'd last been searching for a good facility, the number of people advertising their services as placement specialists had grown considerably. I had been forced to find facilities to tour myself, and to rely on my own judgment and intuition; no professionals fell over themselves to advise me or tour with me. I remember well the half-inch thick list of facilities and homes in Washington State given to me by our caremanager that was my responsibility to peruse. Obviously, the aging-and-dementia business had expanded, spawning new services and specialists.

I hired the placement specialist after just one meeting. She was so warm and generous to me, and so kind to Dad when she evaluated him that I knew immediately she was the one to work with. She was also a nurse and she spent a considerable amount of time talking to him in order to determine his care needs. Later, she told me that during their conversations, Dad would occasionally lean over to her and ask her a questions. "Do you see the snakes?" he asked, pointing to a place on the patterned carpeting. She reported that he would watch her intently as she replied. "Yes, I do see some snakes, right over there! How odd." Her answers seemed to relax him.

It was unclear whether it was a way for him to test whether he could trust her and she was on his side in seeing the same things he did, or if he really wanted to test whether his perceptions were accurate. I know that at other times, he would step exaggeratedly over lines on the carpeting, cautioning me to look out for the stream of water. It was evidence to me of the Lewy body gaining a greater hold in his brain.

She specialized in Adult Family Homes, which are private care facilities, usually in the owner's home. These facilities are licensed by the state and allowed to have only five to six patients at any one time. Having a home environment without the excess noise and activity of a big facility seemed like the way to go. There are many reasons an individual or family may choose to run an Adult Family Home, from strictly financial to a love of helping the elderly. Like many aging and care facilities and services, it is a business often populated by immigrants to the US; we toured many houses owned by Romanian and Filipino families. The type of house differs as greatly as the type of care - some of the houses we toured were large and elaborately decorated, some small and cozy, some small and run-down – and it was obvious that to some owners it was a labor of love, while to others it was a job.

The best thing about an Adult Family Home, in my opinion, was its size. There was a much greater ratio of staff to residents, so Dad would be receiving more personal care. In addition, since they only had six residents, an Adult Family Home would most likely be quiet and not over-stimulating. I was sure that Dad would respond better to calm and quiet environments, with low levels of stimulation and input. Plus, Dad had loved living in his own home and I thought being in a house again would be reassuring for him.

Our professional would choose several homes for us all to tour. Del, especially, would have to approve any new place since he not only knew Dad the best but would undoubtedly be spending a lot of time there. Surprisingly, the homes could be really different in their programs and approach; about the only thing they shared was the fact that they were all home-based and family run.

Although the specialist was aware of Dad's symptoms and behaviors and was locating houses accordingly, I was still concerned that they really wouldn't want to deal with aggression and acting out and wouldn't want to accept Dad. It was the same type of fear I'd experienced the first time I looked for housing – could I find a place that would accept him? It was heightened now because his current facility was, in essence, kicking him out due to behavioral issues. I wasn't even sure how Dad would respond to his impending move since he was much less lucid than the last time I'd moved him.

There were just so many things to worry about, and I hoped that we could find the perfect home for Dad that would meet all his present and future needs, and preclude yet another move. I also intended to find out more about LBD, in hopes that I could help the caregivers keep him happy and comfortable.

*

Frankly, I was just glad I wasn't doing all the work myself this time. I was going through some changes in my own life that precluded having the time and energy to research facilities as I had previously. I had finally been able to evict my ex-boyfriend from my house and was dealing with the paperwork and cleaning tasks that went along with claiming the house as my own. I had also started dating again, something I always seemed to be doing right when Dad was having some sort of crisis or there was some huge alteration to his situation or care.

Things were a little bit different this time around, though. It was five years later and I was five years older. Dating meant possibly having sex with someone new again, which always gives me pause since I am not the most promiscuous person, plus I was now in my late thirties, but I was willing to be open. Fortunately, I felt pretty confident in the looks department, and I felt that even more years of therapy and emotional growth made me a strong candidate, psychologically and emotionally.

I suppose I could have just gotten on with my life without a mate. I could have decided not to risk my heart (and my bank account) again – many people don't, and they live full, rewarding lives alone. I've always been that person who picks herself back up, though, and keeps on trying. I wanted to experience a healthy relationship, and I didn't want to have to care for Dad and myself, alone. But most of all, I believe in love, and connection to other people, and I wanted to see who might be out there for me.

Although entering the dating world once again at the age of thirty-eight was a bit daunting, I was smart enough to want to do it differently this time. Change and upheaval are a normal, if uncomfortable, part of life, and I had to do what so many divorcees, including myself, had done before. I had to re-write what I had regarded as a firm future, reassess what I wanted and needed, and decide in which direction I wanted to go and what kind of relationship I really wanted.

It seemed like the right time to enter a new phase of my life by trying some new things, meeting some new people, and being open to the change that was coming my way. Since I had a bad habit of glomming on to the first decent person I met and calling it a relationship, I knew that I wanted to date many different people. I was also being firm with myself by not expecting, nor hoping, to find "The One" anytime soon. I would force myself to put myself out there as much as possible, accept as many dates as I could, and really look clearly at everyone I met. I would just have to do it in whatever time I had when I wasn't working or looking for places for Dad to live.

I also knew that I had to start doing a lot more research into what Lewy body dementia was and how it would further affect my dad. I have always wanted him to have the most comfortable and safe life possible, and now that I knew there were more kinds of dementia than just Alzheimer's, it seemed like a good idea to investigate as much as I could to make sure that the choices I was making for Dad were the right ones.

A Few Things I Figured Out.

- Do your research! Find out as much as you can about the illness(es) your care receiver may be suffering from. Many of the caregivers I've talked to were the ones who knew that the diagnosis they had wasn't right, so they did the research, spotted the problems, and convinced their doctors of the appropriate diagnosis. I wish I had been more proactive in my research given the differences I saw in Dad. With the changes in health insurance and the decline in number of gerontologists and primary care physicians, more than ever, we are our own best resources and advocates.

- Try to avoid the ER as much as possible since it can be chaotic, confusing, and disorienting for your care receiver. If you have to go, make sure you or another qualified individual is there to advocate. They often give medications that are dangerous for the elderly/people with dementia, and you must be prepared to fight for your loved one. Also, keep a copy of your loved one's chart with you, as well as a list of diagnoses and prescriptions, and make sure you have a current Health Care Power of Attorney or Living Will naming you the decision-maker. I started carrying both Powers of Attorney I had around in my purse and it has saved me trouble more than once.

- The social worker at the ward recommended I request a copy of Dad's entire medical chart for my own records and it was the best advice I'd gotten. He wanted me to have a record of the meds, dosages, and thoughts of the physicians in case I had to protest the actions of the Assisted Living Facility. I highly recommend keeping a copy of every doctor's visit, chart note, prescription, etc., and keep it in one, easily accessible place, along with a list of necessary telephone numbers, a list of prescriptions, and your notebook detailing daily symptoms, behaviors, disease progression, etc.

- I have made mistakes with Dad's care, although some of them were out of my control because of the incorrect diagnosis. There are appropriate medications for people with Lewy body dementia that can calm the behavioral issues and make them more comfortable in their own minds. He might never have had the aggressive incident if on the proper medication. However, I also know that his dementia took the path that it took, and there was no way I could have controlled everything. Knowing the correct diagnosis now has enabled me, I believe, to make his life more comfortable. Learning more about it has enabled me to help other caregivers who are dealing with its symptoms and problems.

- There is more than one kind of dementia. Alzheimer's is the most common dementia syndromes but certainly not the only one. Lewy body dementia, Frontotemporal dementia, and Vascular dementia are also becoming more common - each has its own symptoms and paths of progression. Since they are still massively under-diagnosed, being educated on each one is essential to finding a good doctor and the correct diagnosis. At the onset of illness is when there are the most differences; dementias share the same symptoms later on in the illness progression.

- Be aware that you may need to change care, housing, and medication options for your loved one's optimum comfort. Diagnoses change, needs change, disease symptoms change – everything is possible with dementia. My plan was for Dad to live out his life in one place –and look how that turned out! Be prepared with potential options, or at least names of other facilities that you've liked. Keep up to date files with the names of people or placement companies that can search out housing.

- You may think, or have been told, that a correct diagnosis doesn't matter. It is true that the only firm way to determine these diseases is at a brain autopsy. However, we are learning that the dementias can be really different in terms of medication, choices about surgeries and other care, environmental and housing choices, and behavioral approaches. People with LBD can have severe reactions to many medications, including non-prescription ones. Do your research and double-check with your doctor before administering medication. Keep a notebook recording reactions when a new drug is administered to inform the doctor. I know now that **traditional** anti-psychotic medication, such as Haldol, is contra-indicated for Lewy body sufferers, so he should never have been on Zyprexa. Newer anti-psychotics, called **atypical**, can often be helpful for LBD; drugs like Seroquel and Clozaril. The dementia medication, Exelon, has been shown to be helpful for cognitive and behavioral issues. Anti-depressants may also help an LBD patient, but again, check with the doctor. The LBDA has a glossary of medications on its website that is very helpful. Anesthesia, even for simple operations, has been found to affect dementia sufferers and the elderly in many negative physical ways and should influence any decisions about non-emergency or elective surgical procedures.

- It is also possible to suffer from a combination of different types of dementias; some brains upon autopsy show elements of Alzheimer's and Lewy body, for example. Those suffering from Lewy body tend to live two to eight years after diagnosis. Alzheimer's sufferers can live for fifteen to twenty years, or longer, after diagnosis. Since my father has already lived for at least thirteen years with some form of dementia, we think he probably suffers from more than one kind. We will most likely never know for sure.

14.

True Romance

"There's someone out there for everyone – even if you need a pickaxe, a compass, and night goggles to find them." Harris Telemacher, *LA Story*.

I have said often that when you are a caregiver, nothing's free of dementia - not work, not home, not relationships, not even sex – not when you're living alongside it like most caregivers. Like everything else related to dementia, trying to start a new relationship was a case of: you can do it but it's not going to be easy, and weird things are sure to happen. In fact, on this chilly New Year's Eve day I was late for a date, and thereby belting down a state freeway, because I had been forty miles north of the city, dealing with Dad's care and housing.

We were looking at a lot of different Adult Family Homes in our efforts to find a new home for Dad. Our professional had chosen a particular home for us to tour; unfortunately, the only time we all had available was New Year's Eve day, which felt like an odd day to be looking at Adult Family Homes. Nonetheless, we had all gathered at the house to meet the owners and take the tour; a tour I had just ducked out of early so that I could race to meet my new friend and potential mate. I was anxious I wouldn't make it in time. Once again, caregiving was infiltrating every part of my life.

Every potential relationship would be affected by the fact that I was a caregiver. Since I was still the youngest caregiver I knew, I was doubtful that anybody I met would *also* be a caregiver, so they would have to be very understanding of my role. I realize that at times I have had kind of an odd life, with many events and milestones happening in reverse or not at all, so it is sometimes hard for me to judge what is normal. (I was pretty sure mine was a "non-normal" situation. If there are other caregivers going through something similar I hope this helps!)

I'm fairly certain, however, that there are plenty of men and women out there looking for love in their middle years, and plenty of *them* have something else going on in their lives or their families' lives, even if it's not caregiving. People have diverse and big lives and I hoped that my dates would understand me and my responsibilities. I would be my father's caregiver until his death and it was important that I stay in the area until that time, so I had to find someone who liked Seattle, or who would like it for the next five to ten years. As Dad's illness worsened, I anticipated more hours spent with him and more involvement in decision-making about his health and care so my potential mate would have to be okay with that as well.

*

I ended up meeting a few people off the dating websites that I liked, and Paul was one of them. Paul's profile was a little bit different from the others. First of all, he was a classically trained actor, but, more specifically, he was interested in Stage Combat and Fight Choreography, which I had never really heard of. Apparently, every time a play with some sort of fight in it is staged - like Hamlet, Romeo and Juliet, or everything, apparently, by David Mamet - someone has to create that fight and make sure it is done safely. Paul was that person.

His profile had a similar list of likes and dislikes as the others, things he was looking for in a person, or trying to avoid. It had the same type of picture, although he had a much different look than most of the guys I saw on the site. He was obviously a big, wide-shouldered man, from what I could see in his picture, bald but with a great smile and a nice face. Some of the things he was about, some of his skills and interests, were unique and funny.

He was a theater teacher, of course, but also a self-proclaimed swashbuckler. He had performed as Santa Clause several times at Seattle celebrations, and freely admitted to being a geek. He loved swords, sword fights, most science fiction, and the "Stars" – both Trek and Wars. The thing that really made me laugh was the last sentence of his profile, in which he stated that he "liked hats." I just really liked what I saw, and most of what I saw matched what I was interested in and looking for. He seemed like a really nice guy, we shared a lot of interests, and there had been an evident spark in our exchanges. He was definitely the best result so far to come out of my months of looking. I was hopeful that I had reached the end of my quest.

Once I got to the coffee shop, everything ended up going really well on that first New Year's Eve date. Paul and I spent several hours sitting and talking, long after our beverages had been drunk, and patrons had come and gone. We had a lot of things in common, and a lot to talk about, including my book and various jobs, his current job creating a fight for a play, and my struggles with Dad and his housing issue. He was sympathetic about Dad and offered to help in any way he could, even if it was just to keep listening to my woes, and I could tell he really meant it. As we hugged good-bye and I left, I was already thinking about when I might see him again, and hoping we would talk again.

I knew there was every possibility it could go as badly as some of my other dating experiences of the past few months, but I had hope, because I really liked him. He emailed the next day, inviting me to go with him to a model train show, although the email included a disclaimer citing his awareness that a train show was hopelessly geeky and entailed the risk of me never speaking to him again. He confirmed his strong desire to see me again and promised that he would buy me lunch if I agreed to come.

Personally, I liked model trains and thought it was cute so I agreed and we made plans. It turned out to be an all-day affair, and we had a really good time looking at the tiny dioramas with their tiny trains, and looking through the museum where it was being held. I was pretty sure that I really liked Paul; not only did I feel a definite spark, but he was smart and he made me laugh a lot. I also felt that he was a kind and generous person who would really show up for me; a theory that was tested and proven true on our fourth date.

*

During this getting-to-know-Paul period, Del, my sister, and I had continued to tour potential homes for Dad. I spoke to family after family, met residents, looked at bedrooms and group rooms, and asked the same questions over and over. Did they believe in drugging up their residents? What did they do to keep them active and relatively engaged? Did they know how to deal with the symptoms and behaviors of Lewy body, and what were their care strategies? Did they have twenty-four hour care for when Dad got up in the middle of the night and wandered around?

I was aware that many of my questions and goals had remained the same in the interim between this search and the last one; the new questions were all about how they would deal with the new disease presentation. Finally, it came down to two houses relatively close to each other, both of which we had liked very much. The deciding factor in my mind was the owner of one of the houses, a man named Greg, who would be the main caregiver and who had already had extensive experience caring for men with Lewy body dementia.

He described the residents he had cared for, and how their aggressive and dangerous behavior eventually calmed down and disappeared, all without the anti-psychotic drugs he professed to dislike, and I could feel his compassion and genuine feeling for these poor men. He was not a tall man, but he was fit and well-muscled; it looked like he wouldn't have any trouble managing aggressive behavior, but I could tell that he could be gentle and caring as well.

It was obvious that he and his family, including his shy, kind wife, really loved what they did, and that they excelled at it. We brought Dad to the house for lunch and right away he seemed comfortable and reasonably happy. That was all I needed; we reserved a room for Dad and made plans to move him in February.

I was apprehensive about the move for many reasons, the most important being concern about my dad. He had lived in the same place for three years – his room had become his safe place and his home. He was familiar with the caregivers and they knew him, and he was intimately acquainted with the physical details of the facility. I was uncertain how he might react to such a drastic change in his home, especially since he had declined so much cognitively since the last time I had moved him.

The move, itself, was also causing me some apprehension. I couldn't do it on my own, and I didn't really feel like I could ask any of my friends for assistance - I knew people were busy with their lives, and, let's face it, I've always had trouble asking for help. I was unsure what my sister's schedule was and couldn't be sure she was going to be able to make it, so I was pretty sure it would be me and the furniture, alone, a prospect that caused me some dread. Greg had volunteered his help and his pick -up truck, but it seemed so rude to allow my father's new caregiver, who I barely knew, to move furniture.

I mentioned my troubles to Paul on our fourth date, and to my surprise, he insisted that I let him help, refusing to take no for an answer, joking that it would make a very nice fifth date. I had been pretty sure before his offer that he was a good guy, but after that I knew he was. What kind of person volunteers to help someone they don't know well move their demented Father from the lock-down wing of an Assisted Living Facility to an Adult Family home? Paul was that kind of big-hearted person.

I picked him up two days later at his apartment, and drove him over to the Facility my dad was leaving. Del kept Dad busy in the Common Room while we hurriedly packed what few belongings and pieces of furniture had made it through Dad's residence at the

Facility, which actually wasn't much. We packed clothing and books, a few framed prints and pictures of my sister and I, some desiccated plants, and his toiletries. Halfway through the packing, my sister arrived, and I was pleased to be able to introduce her to Paul for the first time. It didn't take long before our cars were packed full and we headed over to the new house where we unpacked everything we had just packed and laid it out again.

I called Del and had him bring Dad over to the new house, nervous about him settling in and/or acting out because he was in a new place, but he settled in quickly and without a fuss. Every time I spoke to Greg in the next few days, it sounded like he was doing just fine. In the end, Dad had no trouble adjusting to his new home. In fact, I think he felt instantly at home both because he was finally back in a house, and also because it was so much quieter and less over-stimulating then the Facility.

Although it had seemed like another huge challenge, in the end, I had made the right decision. Dad's well-being was paramount, and I had found what seemed like the best place for him. I could only make the same wish that I had made the last time; that this was my father's last move and that we had found his final home. Dad settled in without any problems or sleep disruptions and Greg quickly adopted him as a personal project – helping him work out and stretch daily, and talking with him for long periods of time. For all intents and purposes, Dad was a member of the Adult Family Home family and I was happy to see it.

I couldn't have done it without Paul's help, and I really felt he had gone above the call of duty the whole day. If I had been wondering at all whether he would fit into my odd, dementia-flavored life, this had answered any questions. He had turned out to be a really nice guy – perhaps a keeper. I couldn't help being a little frustrated, however, that I hadn't been able to find this out on a few lovely dinner-and-a-movie dates, like everyone else in the world.

I had hoped for too much in hoping that I would just be able to do an average thing that average people my age do all the time. Who takes a new date to move their demented Father? There seemed to be no way for me to conduct a romantic life, or any life, for that matter, without it intersecting somehow with Dad's life. Once again, any attempt to live my own, age-appropriate, normal stage-of-life life was proving to be unlikely.

*

After the experience of moving my father, Paul didn't run away, which seemed promising, so we continued on in our relationship. We slowly made our way through the pitfalls of dating and getting to know each other. We decided to move in together only five months after meeting, but it felt like the right thing to do. I was struck by how different the relationship was from the one that had gone before it; more grown-up and supportive, less dramatic and uncomfortable.

After meeting my dad on the day we moved him in, Paul came with me several times to visit. Something about Paul's face or extroverted personality attracted Dad and made him respond, even when he was having a withdrawn or uncommunicative day. He always seemed to catch a spark from Paul and begin responding to us. I enjoyed watching Paul's animated face as he spoke to my father and tried to get him engaged with us. It was nice watching the two men in my life together.

On one occasion, we took Dad out for a ride in Paul's 1965 Corvair, which he seemed to enjoy a great deal. After we brought him back we sat around talking and the discussion of different engines and ways to fix them roused something long-forgotten in Dad. He brightened up and came out with a few engine related words of his own, and even seemed to remember that he had once owned his own Corvair. It was always so good to see Dad break through his apathy and withdrawal to connect with us. It made me sad that he was so far gone into his disease that he couldn't really process who Paul was or what he meant to me, but the fact that he enjoyed Paul's company made me happy. He just seemed more engaged when I brought Paul to visit.

When Paul asked me to marry him in the romantic garden of our hotel while on a trip to Kauai, I was excited and certain that I had found the right man and we were doing the right thing. I felt a little emotional, however, as we talked about what kind of wedding we wanted and who would be there, because I knew that no parent of mine would be present. At my first wedding, I yearned for my Mother, but at least I had had my dad, handsome in his tuxedo, to represent both my parents and walk me down the aisle. This time, I would have no parents at all. I felt a deep sadness that both my parents were now, in essence, out of the picture and I was effectively an orphan during what would be one of the happiest times of my life.

Paul and I did pay a visit to Dad to tell him we were getting married, however, during which Paul spoke to him man-to-man, promising to take good care of his daughter. We were both convinced that Dad's eyes sharpened in that moment and that he took in and processed what Paul was telling him. When we repeated our happy news, he even smiled and told us, "Good." It surprised me sometimes when I saw a little bit of cognitive coherency in Dad. I have thought for a long time that he is still somewhat aware of the world around him but that he chooses not to participate in it because it is too painful. Occasionally, he comes back from his long, internal journeys and I see a little bit of the man I knew in his eyes.

I can't know exactly how much he remembers or understands, but parts of him are still there. Dad's reaction to our marriage announcement only strengthened that belief. Although he wouldn't be able to be present at our wedding, I still felt he had given us his blessing. Eight months later, we went back to the same hotel where we had gotten engaged and held our wedding in the same garden. Although neither of us had family present during this precious moment - me by circumstance, Paul by choice - I had my lovely Paul and a few close friends who I considered my family.

When the officiant spoke about family and the presence of our ancestors at such a sacred event, I am pretty sure I felt the presence of my Mother, in the most ephemeral way, and at that moment, I thought of my father and brought him into the ceremony in spirit.

*

As a side note, it has been terribly hard to go through some fairly important life events without much in the way of family. I urge caregivers like me to *find* a family, and get their support during these times. I had my close friends stand up for me at my wedding and it almost – although not quite – made up for having no parents or family there. True family exists in the connections you have with people, and that doesn't just mean blood connections. There is a saying that friends are the family given to you by God; whoever you have, include them in your life.

It is also important to truly feel the grief of being without your loved ones. Don't stuff it down or pretend it doesn't exist – give it room to breathe. Their loss is something that we will have to grieve over and over, as our lives change and events happen. And we are rarely given the grace at the time to know exactly when we will share the last special time or moment with our loved ones. That this may be the *last* time you will hear that particular voice, share that moment, feel that regard. Looking at a picture of Dad during a time we were happy and laughing, I realized, as if for the first time, that I was never going to have him like that again. There are no more long-term hopes, goals, or expectations, there is only this day, this hour, to experience as much as you possibly can of your loved one.

As Paul and I pledged to love and support each other for the rest of our lives, I felt blessed to have been given the opportunity to create another family, one of true friendship and partnership. Against the odds, and after months of dating disasters, Paul and I had found each other, and that was something I wasn't sure would ever happen. And even though I was a lifetime caregiver and my life wasn't entirely my own, Paul took us on – both me and my father - for better and for worse.

A Few Things I Figured Out.

- Care homes, also known as adult family homes, board and care homes, residential care or personal care homes offer personalized service as well as room and board for up to six adults. Homes are typically located in specially retrofitted private houses in residential neighborhoods. These residential homes provide lodging, meal services and assistance with daily living activities. Some adult family homes are run by a single person or married couple who lives in the home with residents. Other homes are operated by commercial entities who hire employees to cover 24-hour shifts. Although some adult family homes may admit people as young as age 18, the average age of residents in these specialized homes for the elderly is between 40-80 years old.

- It is never too late to try to change something about your life. I am living proof that everything can change, just when you least expect it, but that those changes can be positive and life-affirming. Don't let your age, physical condition, responsibilities as a caregiver, or anything else keep you from getting out there and living or learning or finding love, especially if you are young(er) like me. No matter what else is going on in your life, you should make the time to *live* your life.

- It is so important to me to acknowledge the many others who have shared the privilege of Dad's care with me, and without whom I would never have survived. All his caregivers at the Adult day program, Del, and all of the caregivers and staff in each of the places he has called home, have given him personal, loving care. Greg, especially, has been a wonderful caregiver. It is for this reason that I protest when people say that the only good care is in the home by family, because it just isn't true. Dad and I found a family in his caregivers, and their care was good enough for us. There are so many people that can still touch your loved one's life, and from whom they can benefit.

15.

Survivor: Caregiving Edition.

"Many of us follow the commandment, 'Love One Another.' When it relates to caregiving, we must love one another with boundaries. We must acknowledge that **we** are included in the 'Love One Another!' Peggi Speers

I was sitting calmly in the waiting room of a Urology clinic located in a Seattle hospital, waiting for Dad's caregiver, Greg, to bring him to the doctor's office for an appointment. Dad had undergone a double hernia surgery a few months before, and emergency surgery for an infected boil a few months before that. We were meeting today to have a routine follow up with the surgeon. Just as I was starting to realize that it was getting late and I still hadn't seen them walk through the door, I received a call from Greg on my phone.

His usually calm, mildly-accented English was laced with a hint of panic as he informed me that, although he and my father were at the hospital - had, in fact, arrived on time and pulled into the circular front driveway of the hospital in Greg's SUV - they would not be joining me in the nicely appointed waiting room anytime soon. Apparently, as they were five minutes from the hospital, having successfully made twenty-four of the twenty-five miles from the Adult Family Home, Dad said, "Oh, no," and, without any other warning, abruptly vomited all over himself, the front seat, the dashboard, and the floor of Greg's SUV. They had had no choice but to pull into the ER driveway, park, and attempt to address the situation. Greg had called to entreat me to bring whatever cleaning supplies I could obtain so they could clean up.

As I listened, open-mouthed, a weary thought about life as Dad's caregiver popped into my head, and how this job just seemed like it would never end – and never stop surprising me. Until a few minutes before, I had been happy and vomit- free, and now I would have to deal with a problem the magnitude of which was not yet clear, in a public place, without any of the necessary tools or cleaning supplies. For some reason, I was always being caught by surprise by these events. I can only imagine it might be my mind's way of keeping me sane, like the mechanism in women's minds that blurs the memory of childbirth so they'll be willing to go through it again. I repeatedly forget about the crazy-potential of anything involving Dad and his dementia. This must be part of the survival mechanism that helps caregivers cope, otherwise we would have run screaming for the hills and away from our charges years ago.

I hung up the phone and took a few seconds to ponder the situation while swearing vehemently in my head. My only choice of action seemed to be to grab one of the nurses, explain the situation, and receive the cleaning supplies and assistance she or he would no doubt give me. Simple – or so I assumed. One would think, as I did, given the fact that I was currently standing in a hospital, that vomiting would not be an extraordinary event on these premises. That it was a common, even, dare I say, continuous, phenomenon, hardly to be remarked upon, and as such, that the staff would be well equipped to deal with it. Apparently, I was wrong.

The first person I approached was the front desk receptionist. Catching her attention, I explained who I was, reminded her that I had just checked in on behalf of my father, and explained that, while he was technically here for his appointment, he had vomited in his caregiver's car and needed to be cleaned up before being moved. I pleaded for some towels or other appropriate materials she might have to get him cleaned up. For a minute, it seemed like she wasn't even sure what I meant by vomit, and then, for several more minutes, she labored under the misconception that he had vomited somewhere *in* the hospital. She asked me if he had been admitted.

I explained once again that he hadn't been ill IN the hospital, per se, but in the car, which was even then parked downstairs, awaiting my presence, and any cleaning supplies I could scrounge. This still seemed to be a little beyond her grasp, but she agreed to grab a nurse to see what they could offer. Puzzled at how much of a problem this was causing, I watched her head off down a hallway, and that was the last I saw of her for about five long minutes, during which I imagined my poor Dad, surrounded by cold vomit, and Greg, no doubt mildly cursing my continued absence.

I saw her go into and out of several doors and hallways then I saw her stop a nurse and talk to her quietly, after which they both disappeared. I kept waiting for her, or someone, to show up laden with supplies, and I was getting more and more impatient and puzzled at the delay. I was in a hospital, for God's sake, how hard could it be to grab some towels or something. I was also practically jigging with frustration, imagining the scene playing out two floors below me in a Lexus SUV. Finally, the receptionist came back but only to tell me that she was still trying to locate someone to help me. A minute later, a nurse followed her down the hall but as she began to talk to me she seemed to share the same confusion about what had happened and where.

She asked me the same questions about Dad and where he had been sick; in his room? Somewhere in the hospital? Had he been admitted? It was right around this point that I admittedly lost my shit a little. Tensely, I explained once again that he had been in the car with his caregiver, coming here for an appointment which we were now twenty minutes late for, and had vomited while IN the car just as they pulled into the parking lot.

I added, only slightly agitatedly, that they were both waiting there, in the cold, for me to come down to help them so, did they, in fact, have any towels or garbage bags or anything I could take that might help to clean him up? I managed to refrain from adding angrily that, surely, since I was, in fact, standing in a hospital, they must have some means of cleaning up this sort of problem? At this point the fog seemed to lift somewhat and the nurse wandered off to look for some towels, leaving me alone AGAIN, while I got more and more anxious, again imagining poor Greg and Dad downstairs.

A few minutes later, she returned, clutching some small, plastic wastepaper bags, a wet towel, and some rubber gloves, which she pressed into my hands. I stared for a moment at the sheer inadequacy of what she had given me, looked at her, forced out a muttered thank you and began walking as quickly as I could out the door, heading for the front of the hospital.

I was furious at how slow and inept the staff had seemed to be! They had given every impression that this was the first time they had experienced someone vomiting, for all the comprehension they showed about what might be needed. The lack of compassion or assistance infuriated me. I'm sure I looked a little insane, lurching down the hall on my arthritic knees and feet, brow furrowed, jaw set, muttering to myself. I was a little concerned at the paucity of supplies I actually had in my possession and was in no way confident it would be enough to fix the situation. Luckily, I spotted a bathroom on the way: slamming the door open, I attacked the paper towel dispenser and removed as much of the paper as I could carry, grabbing a few black garbage bags out of the can for good measure.

There I was, hustling down a busy corridor of the UW hospital, clutching a wadded bouquet of garbage bags with one hand and latex gloves with the other. I had several towels slung over my shoulder, and paper towels wedged under an elbow like Frankenstein's Bride of Waste Management, lacking only a toilet paper veil to be complete. As I skidded around a corner and irritably dodged tired-looking doctors in white coats and nurses clad in squeaky shoes and Easter egg pastel-colored smocks, I thought about how unequipped to do this job I felt sometimes.

I spotted Greg first, next to his SUV, holding Dad's leather jacket over the sidewalk while gingerly trying to clean it with a fast food napkin. I then glimpsed my poor father through the windshield of the car as he sat in the passenger seat, face set with a miserable, humiliated look. The door was open, presumably to air out the car. Greg looked up and caught sight of me, relief crossing his handsome features as I, clutching my cleaning products, approached him.

I began apologizing as soon as I got within earshot, explaining how apparently inept the staff had been and how long I had waited while they tried to figure out what was going on and what to give me. I held up my inadequate cleaning supplies, explaining that in the end, all they had given me was one wet towel and some garbage bags. My explanation may, or may not, have been laced with expletives, something I usually tried to keep to a minimum around Greg. In fact, he may have looked a little surprised at my language, having never heard me at my full swearing stretch before, but he was gracious as always, and didn't seem to hold my lapse in decorum against me.

He calmed me down somewhat, saying soothingly that he had had some napkins in the car and had made some progress in cleaning up my father, who seemed to be doing a little better. We both turned to look at Dad in that moment, his face miserable, arms slack at his sides, vomit covering him, his seat, and the front dash and carpeting in front of him. Greg clucked sympathetically and began dabbing at my dad with the towel and helping him gently out of his flannel shirt so he could clean it off.

We worked together to get Dad as clean and comfortable as possible, then Greg took a moment and a few paper towels to try to swab out his car. I told him to get it detailed and send the bill to me, since that was probably all that would fully remove the smell. We propped Dad into a handy wheelchair, draped his jacket around him as best we could, and headed into the hospital to get the doctor visit over as quickly as possible.

We had to explain to the doctor what had happened, yet again, while my poor father shivered in only his tee shirt and a thin hospital blanket. Luckily, once he finally grasped the details, the surgeon examined Dad quickly, and we were able to drape his jacket around him once more and get him back in the car. Watching Greg and my father driving off, I reflected on the experience that had just taken place, as well as the medical issues and surgeries that had gone before. It was certainly not the worst event I'd ever lived through with Dad, or the craziest, but it definitely was the last straw. I just felt exhausted by it all; it was hard enough dealing with my *own* medical issues, let alone a long string of unexpected medical issues for my usually-healthy Father.

I'll never know if my poor father was just agitated about being in the car after having just had his dinner, or whether some part of him recognized the place where he had undergone so many painful, uncomfortable events. Maybe he was protesting being there again the only way he knew how – viscerally. It ended up being the last time that Dad left the house. From that moment on, I enlisted a doctor that would come to his Adult Family Home and examine him there, so he didn't have to be agitated or uncomfortable. Hopefully, he will continue on to the end, in relative good health, but I can only hope.

This is my life as a caregiver, an on-going battle between order and chaos, between coordinating my father's life and health and all the crazy things that only seem to happen when you're dealing with any type of dementia. To survive dementia, one has to relinquish a fair amount of control. I have often had to remind myself of this in my tenure as a caregiver. This is just the latest of the ten or so years of care-giving, bill-paying, grief-feeling, choice-making, doubt-suffering moments that have comprised my life. And it is just the beginning of the rest of the unpredictable, possibly unmanageable years to come. To avoid a personal breakdown, it takes a certain amount of surrender to the fact that we can't always control everything that is happening to our loved one, and, by extension, us. However, there are ways to make sure that we survive caregiving.

*

Being a complete novice as a caregiver, without access to support groups or peers, may have caused me to make many mistakes during the course of caring for Dad. However, I also believe it may have allowed me to avoid some of the worst soul-searching, self-shaming, and second-guessing that many caregivers seem to go through. I definitely questioned my decisions and my actions from time to time, and I felt some guilt for some of the things I had to do, but, by and large, I just got on with it. Although I made some sacrifices, emotional and physical, to care for my father, I was pretty selfish from the get-go. As much as possible, I made sure my needs got met equally with his.

As I had contact with more caregivers, I began to get a sense of how complicated the caregiving situation was. Since I had done it largely on my own, without a community, I had just done what seemed best to me at the time and things worked out fairly well. As I took in the stories I was told, as well as blog posts, forum posts, and Facebook comments, my situation began to look more like the exception than the role.

I took note of some of the mental, physical, and emotional challenges that caregivers faced in performing their duties, and the many ways that they beat themselves up, in body and soul, for their actions and decisions. I could see, as have many other advocates and writers, that the type of caregiving most commonly being practiced was a non-sustainable model.

Caregiving by its very nature brings with it impossible choices, unacceptable options, crushing emotions, and dead-end situations (no pun intended.) Taking care of someone with a progressive illness, as most of them are, requires constant action, decision, and movement of some type or another. Running someone's entire life alongside your own is difficult. Watching a loved one succumb to a terrible disease is heart-breaking. Giving up your own precious time and energy on this planet is a sacrifice.

There are so many potential dilemmas and pitfalls that caregivers face. There are often no clear cut choices, no set in stone options, and no absolutes, and we must navigate our way as best we can through the difficulties. There was no one to make any rules or give out guidelines, so people just made it up as they went along using who they were and what they heard, learned, and believed. There is not much official or professional training for the "family" caregiver so most family caregivers are thrust into the job without proper training in how to care for a patient or themselves.

I think that, lacking much official structure and guidance, caregiving has evolved into something toxic and self-destructive. Doctors, advocates, professionals, *and* caregivers, all need to fight what caregiving has become, personally and individually, one caregiver at a time. We must teach people how to survive caregiving; and maybe even win at it.

*

There are a lot of different types of jobs in this world. There are jobs that demand a lot of dedication, both physical and mental. These jobs consume whatever people are willing to sacrifice - time, relationships, energy, and health – but these are generally voluntary sacrifices. Sometimes, people seem to become whatever it is that they do, identifying themselves by their work and position. There are other jobs that require very little in terms of physical or mental exertion; jobs that individuals perform every day and then forget about until the next day. Some people love their jobs, others despise them; some people work to live, others live to work.

I believe, however, that caregiving might be one of the few jobs, other than the priesthood perhaps, where people have come to believe it is appropriate that you *subsume* your Self and needs to the needs of another. Caregivers routinely neglect their own care, both deliberately and accidentally, in the course of caring for their care receiver. They rarely put their needs or their lives first, yet I do not believe that caregiving should involve making the caregiver, their life, and their needs *less important* than a care receivers'.

Private, family caregivers represent an enormous fiscal blessing to a government that would rapidly become insolvent if it had to address all of the growing costs of caring for illness and/or dementia; such as professional, paid caregivers. It is to the benefit of society that caregivers are made to feel that it is "normal" to care for family members and put them first, because we are providing a great deal of necessary unpaid labor. What society, the government, and caregivers themselves, don't yet seem to understand is that caring for another to the detriment of oneself is not cost effective. In fact, it will have far greater costs, both financially and physically, than caring responsibly and selfishly.

There must be more balance involved in what is good for you and what is good for your care receiver, between your needs and your receiver's needs. Otherwise, things will go badly for the both of you. I believe one simple thing, with all my heart, about <u>all</u> caregivers, and it is simply this – that they <u>matter</u> – exactly as much as the person they are caring for. I tell this to every caregiver I speak to, early and often. You, as a person, matter and your life has a value exactly equal to the value of the person you're caring for.

While it's true that, for whatever reason, they are now relying on you and your job is to care for them in the best possible way, please remember that it is still a job: your life, your "self" is important, too. Your "self" includes your spirit, your soul, and all that defines you as a human being. It is the core of who we are and how we define ourselves. It reflects your importance as an individual, that you are vital and unique and that you matter just as much as anyone else on this planet.

As caregivers, we must be given all of the facts, information, and resources. We must be allowed to make our own choices, according to our own limitations, abilities and beliefs, taking into account all the possibilities, without the toxic input of others or of society. Working hard at the job of giving care is a good thing – what is not good is the "normal" expectation that the life and needs of the caregiver should be buried beneath those of the care receiver; the perception that it is the patient who truly matters, not the caregiver. Why should we live with the idea, whether imposed by ourselves or by others that our lives have less value than the lives of those we care for? What caused us to start believing this? I suspect that for many caregivers it is either part of their personalities or a natural consequence of how they were raised.

I know *I* was expected to make many emotional sacrifices for the good of my family. I grew up always with the unspoken expectation that I would be the peacemaker and the caretaker in my family and it is a role I have continued into adulthood. I am the good listener, the friend who will always be there to help and support, the one that cares. I was never encouraged to look after myself first – to be selfish.

The very word, *selfish*, has become such an ugly, pejorative word, signifying that we are choosing our needs first in the most narcissistic fashion. That we are taking up space and resources in a way that is unthinking and uncaring of others. In other words, that we are considering ourselves a human being who matters just as much as the next. We throw the word around so unthinkingly and judgmentally that it has become a bad word in most people's mouths. It has become a word, I think, that is meant to shame us into ignoring our own wants and needs in favor of another's and that we are acting wrongfully and against the social code of conduct if we put ourselves first. I think it is time we reclaimed and redefined this word because I don't think it actually deserves to be a bad word.

I compare it to the word childish, which has negative connotations of immaturity. When you remove the suffix of the word, -ish, and replace it with, "-like", you get childlike, denoting much more acceptable traits. Traits like wonder, imagination, and purity. The word "like" is also positive, meaning to care about or prefer someone or something. Let's replace the suffix on selfish and turn it into self-like, which just represents in a nutshell what we, as caregivers, need to be doing. We need to "like" ourselves enough to put ourselves first, perform self-care, and not feel guilt or shame for our actions and decisions.

I have taken it upon myself to tell every single caregiver I meet how amazing they are, what an amazing job they are doing, and that they matter just as much as their charge. That what they have chosen to do for their loved one is worthy of recognition and praise. And that it is also a challenging, difficult, often overwhelming *job*, not just a pastime or time spent "helping out." I hear the surprise in their voices; surprise at the realization that this might be true, and that someone would recognize it, and recognizing it, name it. Surprise at the thought that they are performing a job that most would choose not to do – and performing it well. But why should this be such a surprise? Why do caregivers not know every day of their lives that they are doing an amazing job? Because we are encouraged so often not to put ourselves first, not to think of ourselves and what we are doing as important – not to be selfish.

Admittedly, the media is increasingly paying lip service to the whole, "care for the caregiver' issue, which is all to the good. Unfortunately, many still seem content with trotting out that oft-used, clichéd story about how when you're on an airplane and the oxygen masks come out, put your own on first before helping others with their masks. The lesson being that you have to care for yourself before anybody else, otherwise you won't be fit to give care – which is a good lesson, there's no doubt. However, when using the oxygen mask story, nobody mentions that air masks only come out when the plane is in trouble and about to crash.

I would like to get to the point where we avoid the oxygen mask situation altogether. We need to really take some action so that caregivers aren't in a position where they even *have* to choose between their own health and well-being and that of their care-taker; i.e., choose which mask to use first. I'd like to convince caregivers to enter into caregiving with the right attitudes and skills. Caregivers believing that their lives and health are valuable and worth maintaining is the place to start, then we add things like support, outreach, and training.

*

We may hear the words, "burn out" and "compassion fatigue" applied to caregiving, but what do these terms really mean? What is burning out exactly, what does it look like and how and when does it happen? The answer is simple: caregivers too often become burned out because they have given too much to their care receiver and have exhausted themselves physically and emotionally. You don't have to be a caregiver to feel burned out and exhausted from job or family responsibilities, political duties, or any other activity or person that demands a great deal of energy and commitment. Allowing oneself to become depleted and exhausted by anything is never a good thing, but it has particularly dangerous ramifications for family caregivers because they have another person's life and well-being in their care.

Like grief, burnout can look like many different things and manifest in a lot of different ways. Excessive anger at a care receiver, friends, family members, or others. Anxiety or obsession about the future. Feeling overwhelming guilt and shame because of actions or decisions. Feeling totally overwhelmed and unable to cope. Depression, inability to care about events or people, as well as irritability, lack of focus and concentration.

Burn out can include exhaustion or fatigue, with possible sleeplessness, health problems, back issues, muscle and joint pain, getting colds or the flu often, eating badly and not exercising. The difficult emotions, harsh realities, repeated stresses, and frequent overextension manifest in a caregiving situation can affect everyone in the relationship – physically, mentally and emotionally.

Caregivers report higher levels of stress than non-caregivers. They also describe feeling frustrated, angry, drained, guilty or helpless as a result of providing care. Studies show that close to 16% of caregivers feel emotionally strained and 26% say taking care of the care receiver is hard on them emotionally. 3/5 of caregivers aged 19-64 reported fair or poor health compared with only 1/3 of non-caregivers. One in ten caregivers report that their duties have caused their physical health to worsen. 30% of caregivers report that they do not go to the doctor as often as they should.

Caregivers suffer from increased rates of physical ailments – headache, exhaustion, persistent bouts of cold and flu, chronic pain, and back pain. They also have an increased tendency to obesity and development of serious illness such as auto-immune diseases, heart disease, diabetes, and cancer – caregivers have a 23% higher level of stress hormones and a 15% lower level of antibody responses. Studies also consistently report higher levels of depressive symptoms and mental health problems among caregivers than among their non-caregiving peers; between 40 to 70% of caregivers have clinically significant symptoms of depression, with approximately one quarter to one half of these caregivers meeting the diagnostic criteria for major depression.

Depressed caregivers are more likely to have coexisting anxiety disorders, substance abuse or dependence, and chronic disease. A study found that one in four caregivers have contemplated suicide more than once a year – one-third said it was likely they would attempt it. Studies also show that both caregiver depression and perceived burden increase as the care receiver's functional status declines which translates as higher levels of clinical depression being attributed to people caring for individuals with dementia. Sadly, 30% of caregivers *pre-decease* their care receivers. Burn out is a serious condition!

*

I have nothing but empathy for full time, family caregivers devoting most of their time and energy to another. Caregivers who are dealing with the physical issues and challenges of their care receivers by administering medication, caring for ailments and injuries, and dealing with the breakdown of physical systems. Caregivers who are weathering behavioral issues, and providing care, feeding, and entertainment to increasingly challenged individuals. They are most likely also managing difficult and complex medical, governmental, legal, and financial issues and dealing with the corresponding institutions and entities.

We all know that inanimate, mechanical systems require regular maintenance and do not benefit from overuse or strain, which can cause the mechanism to fail or break down. Operators follow basic guidelines of care to prevent system failure. Why as caregivers are we so reluctant to admit that the same basic guidelines might also apply to us? That we are a mechanism in need of proper maintenance. Physically speaking, you have to take care of the tool that is essential to the job – in this case, you.

It is far too easy to burn out as a result of the immense obligations that the job requires. Caring for another is usually long term, often physically challenging, and always emotionally draining. If you let the hardships of caring affect your ability to care safely, if you lift with your back and not your knees, so to speak, then you won't be able to stay the course. The first duty of a caregiver is to go on caring, and this must include caring for oneself, otherwise your charge will be left without a caregiver, and you will be of use to no one, including yourself.

I'm not saying all of this to shame caregivers or make them feel like this is one more area of their lives that needs time and energy put into it. I understand that caregivers often have limited resources, that they may not have anyone else able or willing to help them, and that they may be working full-time then caring for their loved one, as well as a host of other family and life obligations. It may seem as if there is no other way to do everything that needs to be done other than to run the mechanism full tilt and flat out every day, without thought of the repercussions. The problem is, that there will be repercussions – serious ones – physical and emotional.

There are so many difficult emotional and mental elements to the burden of caregiving that contribute to worsening compassion fatigue. 13% of caregivers feel frustrated with the lack of progress made with the care recipient. In other jobs, discernible and quantifiable progress or improvement is usually made. An illness bad enough to require full time caregiving usually leads to decline and death, regardless of how hard the caregiver works or cares. This can be difficult to adjust to in our society of measurable achievement and striving for improvement.

Caregivers are watching the physical and mental failure of someone they love and seeing them endure those losses. They are facing the loss of that loved one while dealing with, possibly negative, emotions and actions of friends and family members. They are having to curtail and compromise their own lives, including family and personal growth, while dealing with the stress of managing the lives of their loved ones as well as their own. Is it any wonder that caregivers are feeling fatigue?

Emotionally speaking, the signs of caregiver compassion fatigue can often be more subtle than the physical. A feeling of being overwhelmed, anxiety about present and future events, irritability, sudden rage, and lack of concentration are common internal responses and can be very damaging to the caregiver's health and well-being. Some caregivers may start to feel isolated or alone or as if nobody understands or is helping. Other caregivers may feel sad or apathetic about events or self-care. These are all natural emotional responses that have become exacerbated by fatigue and stress.

One of the most common and dangerous emotional responses can be depression. We've all felt sad or depressed, sometimes for extended periods of time. Feeling depressed can be a normal reaction to loss, life's struggles, or an injured self-esteem. But when feelings of intense sadness - including feeling helpless, hopeless, and worthless - last for many days to weeks and keep you from functioning normally, your depression may be something more than sadness. It may have slipped over into clinical depression, which can have negative implications for both caregiver and care receiver.

Caregivers often feel rage or irritation at their care receivers and may resent their constant neediness. Strange impulses may pop into their minds. Caregivers may at times hate their charge or feel as if they want to secretly hurt or dispose of their charge. They may wish that something would happen to their loved one, or that they would die. Exhausted caregivers often snap and lash out at their charge verbally then later beat themselves up for it. These actions and emotions are then allotted an outsized importance by the overloaded brain of the perpetrator, piling stress on top of stress, grief on top of grief, which can ultimately lead to depression and other dysfunctions if it hasn't already.

Everything that caregivers feel are normal and appropriate to the burdens and stresses of caregiving. What is not appropriate, of course, is acting on them to the point of injury – verbal or physical abuse. Although people still don't want to talk about it, elder abuse is unfortunately very common due to the difficulties of the job, the exhaustion, and the emotions involved. Statistics show that spouses who are at risk of depression and are caring for a spouse with cognitive issues are more likely to engage in harmful behavior towards their care receiver.

When I got the phone call from Greg about my father being sick in the car, I'm sad to say that my first response was aggravation with Dad. I just didn't have the energy to deal with drama that day – it had taken enough energy for me to get to the hospital after a morning's work. If I had been the only one caring for the situation, I'm pretty sure I would have been snappy and irritated at my poor father, while I dealt with a situation that took energy from me. I am fortunate in that I had Greg there to help me deal with it and to take Dad home after the appointment, so that *I* could go home and rest. Most family caregivers don't have that option.

If as a caregiver you don't value yourself and your needs, and you don't take steps to make sure they are taken care of, it will definitely be reflected in the quality of care you provide your loved one, leading to unhealthy expectations, anger, resentment, and, possibly, abuse. When a tense or dangerous situation arises, caregivers need to place their loved one somewhere safe and secured, where they cannot hurt themselves, and leave them alone. Walk away before you *do* away with your care receiver. I'm generally against over-medicating, but if a physician has prescribed sedatives or some other calming agent, don't hesitate to use them. Call a friend or family member and ask them to take your place for a brief time. In other words, ask for help.

*

While I never had the urge to physically or verbally abuse my father, I know there were times I felt intensely angry at him. I only cared for him part time, but even that, paired with my chronic illness, was enough to make me feel at the end of my rope when I lived with him. There were days when I had had enough of his moodiness or depressed affect, or just his neediness; on those days, I left him in the living room with a magazine and I shut myself in my room with a funny DVD. Dad also visited an adult day care program once a week that gave me a few hours off to do much-needed errands or take care of business affairs. I also made sure to take a short break during the day if I was starting to feel irritated or overwhelmed.

I did feel a little emotionally overwhelmed by the fact that I was grieving at this terrible thing happening to someone I loved, as well as at the loss of a father figure. I was angry that he had gotten sick in the first place, and that I was the one left to care for him. I struggled with resentment of my father, throughout the years I was physically caring for him. Not only did I resent having to care for a man who didn't care for me in childhood, I was angry at what I perceived to be his escape from the mess he had left behind; emotional, clerical, medical and financial. I felt it had been left up to me to clean up a mess in which I had no part, and I sometimes begrudged every single bit of energy that it took.

Resentment alone is a powerful and exhausting emotion that will affect the quality of the care you give, as well as the attitude of your charge. Your care receiver will feel it if you are angry with or resent them and it will cause a lot of pain and discomfort to both of you. And my father could always tell when I was feeling emotional towards him; he could feel it physically, even though he didn't understand intellectually what was happening, and it could cause him to withdraw or even act out. Care receivers often take their emotional cues from their caregivers; they pick up on moods and attitudes and it influences their mood and behavior.

I have heard from his current caregivers that if they are impatient or irritated when dealing with him, he will react with irritation and stubbornness, refusing to do what they want. How often have you snapped at your charge or been irritated by something they did, only to have them act out for the rest of the day or be upset for hours? If you are reasonably rested, happy, and calm, it's a pretty sure bet that your charge will be as well – yet another reason to put some of your own needs first.

For the most part, I was able to deal with my feelings through therapy, where I had the freedom to express all of my feelings and learn appropriate ways to manage and soothe them. I could tell my therapist all of my nasty thoughts and icky feelings without shame or judgment. Going through the emotions in her presence took the charge away from them. Anytime I read a memoir by a caregiver who shared at least some of my experiences and emotions, I felt better. Every time I read an on-line forum now, or a blog, where caregivers are being honest about their nasty feelings, I rejoice because I have had those feelings, too!

I think it's vital that caregivers know that other caregivers have had the same mean thoughts and tired impulses that they have had. There is such a strong stigma in our society against emotional dysfunction, distress, and disclosure that it keeps people from being honest about the mental and emotional effects of caregiving. It can be hard to know if other caregivers are going through the same uncomfortable experiences, which leaves individuals feeling isolated and possibly ashamed and abnormal.

Caregivers need to hear more about other caregivers and what they have done to survive. Caregivers need to know that it is okay to put themselves first and take care of their own health and life, and why, and what can happen when they don't. This is where support groups and on-line forums can be so helpful because they make public all of those negative feelings and reactions.

Giving care can be hard enough on its own without twisting it from giving from a place of love to one of dysfunction; it is essential that caregivers have the proper emotional support so that they can remain in a place of love. We must take steps to assist those caregivers who feel as if they are on the edge, or who may have already gone over.

Caregivers are both notorious for, and truly gifted at, setting impossible expectations for themselves. They battle personal, and probably unwarranted, guilt and shame, as well as the judgments, projections, and opinions of others. They and the people around them, question their choices, their actions, their motives, their feelings, their integrity, and their hearts; second-guessing actions and reactions – such as placing loved ones in facilities, medicating loved ones, accepting respite care, and feeling anger and resentment towards loved ones. They feel guilt about what they do, what they don't do, why they're doing it, and how they do it. We spend far too much time worrying about what *might* happen or what others *might* think, and feeling guilt and shame about the choices we make, the actions we take, and even about the things beyond our control.

Where do the internal voices of guilt, shame, and worry come from? The ones that tell us to give up so much of ourselves, or that only one way is the right way, or that if we don't control everything, it will all fall apart, or even that we should feel guilty for wanting to live our own lives? Expectations of specific results, self-doubt, self-blame, shame, and guilt can only add to the emotional burden of giving care to a loved one.

Worry, guilt and shame are empty emotions, and yet we are so very good at inflicting them on ourselves. Negative thoughts and feelings can be insidious, exhausting, sneaky, ineffectual, and ultimately, harmful. How much are we wearing ourselves down by carrying these burdens? It can be so difficult to find a way through the difficult feelings, the duties and responsibilities, and the needs and expectations of others. Caregivers are, unfortunately, often prone to feelings of despair, guilt, shame, depression, low self-esteem and self-worth, which sap strength and energy and make contemplating a full life difficult.

However, it is possible to have a life for yourself, both practically and emotionally, while giving care to another. One way to start is by showing ourselves the same empathy we show our loved ones. We must make sure that we are caring for ourselves and placing ourselves and our lives equally alongside that of our care receiver. Empathy with our needs and limitations is essential because our lives are just as important as our care receiver's. Learning how to work with the feelings instead of being at their mercy is crucial to success as a caregiver and survival as a person.

*

There are many ways to give care and many ways to be a caregiver. There is no right or wrong approach or attitude or perspective, no matter what others say. One must give care according to the dictates of the individual situation and one's beliefs, abilities, and limitations. I even support someone *not* giving care if that is what is in their best interest. If you do become a caregiver, it helps to find that which will give us the strength to make it through, whatever that might be, whatever anyone else's opinions or beliefs are. Finding a meaning behind a challenge such as dementia and caregiving can be a good way of adjusting emotionally.

Sometimes it is easier if we can relate a challenge to some larger pattern. We can believe tests are sent by God or Divinity, for some unknowable purpose, to allow us to show our courage and devotion, resulting in some afterlife reward. Some decide blessings come to us when we are ready or when we are most in need. Others feel that the Universe is either random in its blessings and challenges, or even that it is malicious, waiting until the worst moment to strike out. I have had a lot of challenges in my life and I have to admit that my beliefs hover somewhere between believing it's all about the journey and that blessings come when we need them, and that the Universe is random.

Some caregivers claim the burden they've been given is a blessing, or a chance to fulfill marital or filial vows. For some, it is a chance to spend quality time with their loved one, or a way to pay back all the love and care given over the years. Some may seek to forgive their loved ones or find forgiveness during this struggle. There are also caregivers who are performing out of duty, or who don't choose to find an enlightened purpose in the challenge of caregiving, who are just doing what they need to do. It is just as likely and acceptable that there is no greater meaning for them than that this is a random bad thing that has happened, and that this is the right thing for each person to be doing, and that this is the way they need to do it.

If we choose, I believe that we can make something bigger and better out of caregiving. I believe we can use it to heal ourselves and our loved ones, to find or give forgiveness, to change a relationship's status quo. We can take our place as a caretaker of our loved one's soul, responsible for everything our charge is and was, as they continue along their lonely road of illness. We can help them along that road. We can't control or fix the situation for our loved ones – we can't take away their pain and fear – but we can be present with them as they experience it, and we can help them live whatever life they have left to them, in the best way possible. We can help them feel the humanity still inside themselves.

There is a phrase in the yogic tradition – "Namaste" – that, roughly translated, means "I see the God in you." I believe there is divinity in everyone – humanity, a certain spirit, a soul. The most basic need of all people, no matter the situation, is to maintain that humanity, to feel as if one is still a human being, and that one still matters. As caregivers, we can see the divine in the person we care for, whatever shape the divine takes for us, and remind them of it, as well.

We just have to make sure we are including ourselves in this – that we are seeing our own divinity. I haven't always been able to find meaning behind having to care for Dad and his dementia. There have been, and still remain, times full of anger and resentment at the hands I've been dealt, and although I think of myself as a fairly resilient and emotionally mature person, it has not always been an easy thing to pick up the cards and continue to play.

*

Don't let an over-loaded caregiving situation go so far and get so out of balance that it is YOU who are in need of a caregiver. I realize that people can achieve some amazing things if they have to; struggling on with duties for years with a debilitating illness or injury. Most people can endure a bad situation for a long time. I know this personally, having had to hack out some sort of real, normal life for myself through twenty years of illness, and ten years of managing Dad's life and care. What kind of life does that lead to, however? Where is the ultimate reward in that behavior? What will happen to the people who are depending on us for so much, if we break ourselves in their service? Who is that really serving?

There is a level of personal accountability that caregivers must admit to and attempt to reach. Compassion fatigue and burn out is nothing to be ashamed about. It can happen to the best of us, we've all had our moments, and it is not a negative reflection on our abilities, dedication, or love for our charge. It just means we are taking on too much. We must believe that being a good caregiver does not involve destroying our bodies and minds. This job can be performed without burning ourselves out and we need to start being truthful about what we can and cannot do, and whether we are coping. We must be responsible for our own mental health and well-being and examine ourselves regularly for some of the more common symptoms of burn out.

If we can begin to recognize the symptoms and problems of compassion fatigue, we may be able to prevent them from even happening, or, at least, catch them earlier. We can then move on to ways to improve the care we give so that nobody, including ourselves, loses out or has to sacrifice more than is safe. We also need to start being honest about our feelings, our situations, and our limitations and about what illness, dementia, and care for another does to families, relationships, and the self. That honesty can help lead us to empathy – for ourselves and our care receivers – that is one of the strongest supports in the long struggle that is caregiving.

For some caregivers, asking for help is the equivalent of severe torture – an admission of weakness. For others, hearing they need to put themselves first may be too touchy-feely and emotional. There are many caregivers who swear that they are the only ones who can provide the best care to their loved ones; an assertion that is patently not true. They are the ones placing an impossible burden on themselves and unhealthily placing their needs below their care receiver's.

Some caregivers don't want to hear advice from anyone who hasn't been right where they are, in exactly the same difficult situation. It's so easy to feel that people outside of the caregiver experience just don't understand, or don't know what they're talking about, and it's true that many of them don't, although I'm pretty sure that being worn out, stressed, and overloaded is a condition that most people understand, despite the cause.

I know it can be really annoying to have people glibly tell you that you need to be selfish, to take more time for yourself, or, that you just need to ask for help! However, I'm inside of the caregiving experience and I can assure you it is possible. It might take some planning, effort, and more asking for stuff than you're comfortable with, but anything is possible. Regardless of where it comes from or how you are able to hear it, the real, basic message remains the same and is valid - you can't take care of someone else if you have broken down. You do have a choice. Sometimes the choice is between something bad and worse, but there is almost always a choice.

Ask for the help you need, whether physical or financial; ask for the financial, physical, or mental support you need to do the job. Unfortunately, not all care-takers can afford to pay their caregiver due to a limited income or reliance on disability and pensions. Sometimes, even if there is enough money, caregivers hesitate to ask for compensation for their time and energy. There can be an expectation that they should provide care out of love or duty, which is a good place to start, but everyone deserves recompense for their time and energy. If money is not available, some other type of exchange might be possible: living rent-free with a care receiver; sharing groceries; or being given the use of a care receiver's car.

There are more organizations than ever, on-line and brick and mortar, aimed at supporting caregivers. Cities and counties are providing increased respite resources as well as social workers who can help with financial, legal, housing, and medical issues. There is more training available now, thankfully, at area hospitals and senior centers, teaching caregivers how to lift properly, perform health care, and deal with a care receiver's emotional issues and behaviors.

Other members of the family might also be willing and able to contribute – either with money, time, or help with responsibilities. There is a vital energy exchange that needs to occur to maintain balance in the relationship - without it, resentment and anger grows and burning out almost becomes a given. Somehow, caregivers must find a way to win back the self-worth and self-value that they may have lost in giving care. You must find the ways that will help you survive and, possibly, thrive.

Interestingly, learning how to be more selfish may have positive repercussions in other parts of a caregiver's life. Developing improved self-esteem and a better sense of self is never a bad thing and can lead to taking better care of oneself physically and emotionally. It could mean escaping a difficult or harmful situation. It could even mean cutting people out of one's life who are draining or non-supportive of personal growth. Developing improved self-awareness could lead to better job, housing, or educational opportunities, or rediscovery of important goals or dreams. Developing an awareness of one's own value as a human being is the path to a better life. We are all of value and we all deserve to live.

Caregivers must start being really honest about where they are in terms of self-care, and whether they might just be heading towards a tiny, little breakdown. It is imperative that we create a new caregiving paradigm – it is imperative that caregivers become more self-like so that they can survive the challenges and tests of caregiving. It might be hard to believe, but I feel that it is actually *the* most caring and responsible thing you can do for your charge; not just physically but emotionally, as well. Then, if we are given the proper resources and tools, such as good wings, maps, and landing gear, we may avoid getting to the point of crashing.

A Few Things Figured Out.

- Selfish is not a four-letter word. Recognize that you have just as much value as a human being as your charge. You are important; take your own needs into account. You must believe that you matter. Being selfish doesn't mean neglecting your charge, it means *not* neglecting yourself - your needs are just as important as your caretaker's. Plenty of people believe that you have to be naturally unselfish to act unselfishly, so they try to make themselves feel something they just don't feel. I believe that's just another way to brainwash us into giving up what we want or need for another. Be selfish! Be self-like! You can still give good care even if you're not Florence Nightingale. You just have to be honest with yourself that sometimes you really hate what you have to do.

- Physical and emotional signs of compassion fatigue, in general: Excessive anger at your care receiver, friends, family members, or others. Allowing yourself to become isolated or withdrawing from friends and family, and an inability to care about events or people. Anxiety or obsession about the future. Feeling overwhelming guilt and shame because of your actions or choices. Feeling totally overwhelmed and unable to cope. Exhaustion or fatigue, with a possible concurrence of sleeplessness. Irritability, lack of focus and concentration. Health problems, back issues, muscle and joint pain, getting sick often, eating badly and not exercising. All of these things, and more, can signify you may have pushed yourself too far.

- Depression can be a realistic reaction to overwhelming stress. Clinical depression requires feeling at least five of the following symptoms at the same time: a depressed mood during most of the day; fatigue or loss of energy almost every day; feelings of worthlessness or guilt almost every day; impaired concentration, indecisiveness; markedly diminished interest or pleasure in almost all activities, nearly every day; recurring thoughts of death or suicide; a sense of restlessness or being slowed down. Depression can lead to things like car accidents, falls, forgetting things and being absent minded. Be careful of society's message that depression is shameful, or your fault, or that it is something you can "get over." Clinical depression requires, and deserves, the intervention of a physician. If you need to take medication to feel better, do it!

- Giving care can lead to feelings of powerlessness, anger, grief, and resentment. Having someone consistent to talk to is important, to help you work out ways of feeling more empowered and in control. Be honest and straightforward, where appropriate, about the circumstances of your life as a caregiver. Ask for what you need, and be patient with those who are unsure how to act. Those who don't give care often don't understand the difficulties and may not offer help - others may not know *how* to help. It is up to us to suggest what we need and how others can help. Help friends and acquaintances help you by being upfront about changing behaviors, needs, and other ways that things will be different.

- Assess the human resources around you. Have you truly explored the ways that others can help you? Are you too proud to ask for help, or are you waiting for others to offer? You might want to rethink these positions. In many cases, people want to help but don't know how. Grab friends, relatives, and anyone who has ever offered help and be specific about what they can do for you: they might not be able to care for your care receiver long-term, but they could sit with them for a few hours while you run errands or take a break; ask for meal help, have people drop off frozen dishes or pick up groceries; ask friends to come over and watch movies; ask friends to do a few of your errands while they are running their own. There are many possibilities if you use your imagination.

- Caregivers deserve, and must sometimes insist on, empathy from others; people who may or may not be directly connected to a caregiving situation but who may feel the need to have an opinion about it. Too often, a caregiving situation can become something of an open forum for the public; perhaps because of its deeply emotional elements as well as the fact that it can happen to anyone. Caregiving can become a polarizing issue but no one else can be a better judge of your situation, abilities and limitations than you; in fact, no one else is *allowed* to be a better judge of these things than you.

- While the impending dementia and changed needs of a loved one is a terrible thing to have to contemplate, it can also be a powerful tool for self-awareness, and self-growth if you so choose. Keep in mind, however, that we have enough problems without worrying about whether we're doing everything right, or doing the right thing, or creating the most meaning, or undertaking the best spiritual journey.

- Worry, as a pastime, actually accomplishes nothing; it is a pointless waste of energy and emotion, better used elsewhere. The antidote to worry is decision and action, even if it is small and careful. If there is a problem, look at the options, make a decision, take some action, and let it go. Guilt can be useful in small doses, if it helps you to follow your moral compass, but it mostly functions as a self-torture device along with shame. Neither of these emotions helps us achieve anything or spurs us to action, they are just emotional burdens we carry that wear us out and make us feel bad about ourselves. If you are clear about your needs and wishes and don't accept guilt, shame, or family pressure you will not make choices you don't feel are right for you.

- Caregiving overload may bring up unexpected impulses; try to become aware when some sort of respite from your care receiver is urgently needed. This can come in the form of taking a personal time out, putting your charge to bed, medicating them, asking a friend to take your place for an hour or two, or calling a professional respite organization. Respite care, whether for a day or a week, is essential for self-care and survival. Don't be ashamed of the fact that you may need respite care, support, or help. This does not signify a failing in your care or dedication, it just means you are human. There are many excellent respite care facilities and adult daycare programs.

- If you have to continue working in addition to giving care, be proactive. The most important tool people in this situation have is communication. Letting employers in on your secret is essential in order to develop a plan of support. Employers will most likely comprehend that an employee with fewer demands and more support will have fewer sick days and be more productive, even if it has to be over a longer period of time. Learn your company's leave policies by consulting your HR department or employee handbook. Know your rights in regards to the Family & Medical Leave Act. Inquire about flex time (the possibility of working from home once or twice a week so you can also perform your care giving duties) and don't abuse work time (do work while you're at work instead of using it as care giving time). Stay organized. Seek help from coworkers and express your gratitude.

- You know the drill! Take care of yourself physically and eat a well-balanced diet with lots of protein, fruits and vegetables, and whole grains. Try to exercise several times a week and get adequate rest. Seek professional help to help you with your feelings and struggles. Keep on top of your own health issues and don't allow them to be ignored. Explore community resources or ask friends how they might be willing to help. Explore yoga, meditation, or other relaxation techniques. Write about your feelings; start a blog or Facebook page. Attend a support group as often as needed and try to get out of the house at least once a week; social activities can help you feel connected and may reduce stress. Give yourself a treat once a month like a haircut, massage, or movie. Stay in touch with friends and family, by computer or phone if necessary. Look to faith-based groups for support and help. Take one day at a time. Learn to set mental priorities.

- All statistics from Family Caregiver Alliance, *Caregiver Health.*

16.

The Right Tools for the Right Job.

"If you ain't got no axe, you cain't cut no wood." John Eaton

One has to have the right tools to cope with the craziness, the unpredictability of our care receivers and the actions and reactions of others. There is help to be had, however, tools for navigating these new experiences of caregiving that will assist you and your care receiver. There are ways to deal with the stress, the strange behaviors, and the complete refusal by a care receiver to do what is in their own best interest. There are ways you can help them, guide them, and keep them comfortable and happy – while also maintaining your own sanity. Keep in mind that to do this, you may have to make uncomfortable choices, choices that others disagree with or complain about. You may have to act in ways that go against your natural inclinations or ideas of normal or moral behavior. Our own behaviors can become our best tools – patience, compassion, imagination - as can our bodies and our minds, as well as outside instruments such as respite care.

The first and best tool in our toolbox is the willingness to be relaxed and open to what our care receiver thinks is reality. I made it a point from the beginning never to try to keep Dad in *my* reality: I met him in whatever time, place, or story he happened to be caught up in and never tried to correct him or remind him of *actual* reality, which used to be common practice - keeping dementia sufferers "reality oriented" which is just unimaginable to me. Who cares whether they think it is 1939 or call you by the name of their long-dead sister? I remembered my aunt, firmly telling my grandmother that she was wrong, that the year was actually different, and that she wasn't talking to the person she thought she was talking to. I questioned it even then, in my early twenties, because it seemed so pointless.

When Dad thought my mother had died giving birth to my sister, I let him think it. When he was sure he had been caught in a storm on his boat and nearly died, I listened and said how fortunate that he survived. I really tried not to ask him questions or talk about things I didn't think he would remember, or that might agitate him because he had made an association I didn't know about. It would only have caused him more anxiety and confusion if I had questioned him about a topic or memory or tried to tell him something he believed wasn't true.

We know that the mind of an individual with dementia has stopped storing new information - factual content is not registered, only feelings. In other words, the camera of their mind has stopped taking current pictures. There are only blank spaces when they try to retrieve memories of the present moment, whereas there are plenty of images of the past in their "photo album." When someone tries to get a dementia sufferer to retrieve factual information that they won't have, they are likely to interpret what is happening in the present through their memories of the past. They will access a different, older memory and try to act on it, causing them to be outside the current reality of the people around them. In addition, it can cause anxiety and confusion because they know they should have those memories but don't know why they don't.

I can't imagine trying to interpret an event, a person, or a conversation of the present through the only tools and maps I had left – pictures and experiences from the past. I, too, would act and sound confused if someone asked me whether I had seen a particular person lately and the only picture I could access was a long-dead sister. Many environments or situations are easily recognizable or decipherable to those of us firing on all cognitive cylinders – even places we have never seen before, we can usually identify as restrooms, hospitals, libraries, or train stations. Lacking those cognitive abilities, it would be like being picked up and placed in an entirely alien land, with no cultural, visual, or linguistic context and being forced to figure it all out and communicate.

Dementia sufferers have been known to confuse doctor's waiting rooms with airport terminals, for example, thinking they were going to be traveling. It seems like a good guess to me, especially if they had traveled a lot: there are a lot of people sitting and waiting, a desk with people behind it and others waiting in line in front of it – makes sense. No wonder frustration and strange behaviors are the norm with dementia. Even when what Dad believed was hurtful to me, I didn't argue with him about it. When I was cleaning out his room, I found a note he had written, one of many that he used to remember events and people. The note averred that I was stealing from him, that he didn't know why I was always in the house, but that he didn't trust me.

One part of the note was a reminder to have his aide help him find a lawyer to rescind the Power of Attorney document I had (something he *did* remember) and get a document that would protect him. This was a really hard thing to read, considering that I was giving him my time and energy, but confronting him with a note he probably wouldn't remember writing, about a subject he probably wouldn't remember contemplating, would have been pointless and agitating.

Other caregivers I have talked to also subscribe to this approach. They find nothing wrong in participating in a past memory with their loved one, knowing that they are being kind and supportive, and that their care receiver is not becoming agitated or being made to feel at fault. They have become masters at engaging with their loved one in whatever space and time seems to be happening.

I also had a different kind of relationship with my father then perhaps most daughters. We weren't close, we didn't really have the traditional established father/daughter relationship, and I wasn't hoping or expecting him to do or feel things he had "always done." I didn't really have to make the "shift in thinking" that I counsel other caregivers to make – or at least, not very often. I found that when I let my heart, my gut, and my instincts lead, Dad and I managed just fine.

It's not hurting anything to let them be content in their minds; in fact, it has been shown to be *more* hurtful, confusing, and agitating for them to be constantly jerked into reality. There are many books now on the market detailing new behavioral approaches on dealing with this issue. These methods advocate meeting your loved one wherever they are, and using what information they are giving you as a way to help and soothe them.

This willingness to be flexible with reality and the truth is part and parcel of another tool that caregivers have – a tool that has proven to be controversial – lying. The use of misinformation, small untruths, distraction, and the above-discussed tool of allowing someone with dementia to believe in a different reality – to make your care receiver happier and more comfortable, and your life a little easier.

*

Lying to a care receiver has become a very prevalent and polarizing issue. Caregivers and family members struggle constantly with the issue of lying to their care receivers. Is it disrespectful? Is it wrong? Caregivers call it "white lies" or "fiblets," or "therapeutic lying" and argue that it makes the struggle of caregiving just that much easier. Other caregivers eschew the white washing, call it lying, and consider it a bad idea, and that the care receiver will know on some level that you are lying, and will cease to trust. The debate rages on, sparking arguments on forums about issues like trust and respect, arguing that our care receivers will know on some level that they can't trust us if we lie, or that we must treat them with the humanity and respect they deserve.

Personally, I feel this issue is being given life and energy that could be better used elsewhere but I can understand the discomfort and distress that motivates the discussion. As a society, I would argue that we already feel ambivalent about lies and lying, so it's no surprise that we project our ambivalence onto the act of caregiving. We would like the subject to be straightforward and black and white; honesty is moral, lying is immoral. Unfortunately, there are too many exceptions to the rule – times when telling the truth would be immoral and destructive, for instance. There are, therefore, a lot of mixed messages around the subject.

As children, we're taught that lying is wrong and we're reprimanded if we do it and rewarded if we don't. It is not long, however, before we start to realize that lying is not a black and white subject. We realize through observation and experience that there exists a moral gray area around lying; there are so-called "white lies," which are apparently acceptable in some situations but are usually unsatisfactorily explained by our parents, who are probably struggling with their own moral relativism. Apparently, there are lies, and there are lies.

This was not really a topic to which I gave much thought, however, until I experienced life with dementia, which caused me to develop my own brand of moral relativism. Personally, I don't care for lying and I strive to be as honest as I possibly can be. However, I tend to think in terms of gray areas anyway, not in blacks and whites, and I know that there may be times when any moral rule needs to be reassessed.

There were times when I realized that maintaining a strict adherence to the truth, or sharing every single fact or detail about an uncomfortable situation, held little moral value, and could, in fact, be harmful. I found it necessary to develop relatively flexible views on lying, honestly, withholding information, and embroidering on the truth when dealing with Dad and his dementia – and I saw nothing wrong with that.

I suppose I lied every time I allowed Dad to wander in his delusions and illusions without the 'truth' being imposed. However, I had to ask myself whether encouraging the cognitively-impaired to believe in a false yet comforting memory was lying, and, if so, whether it was wrong. Would I be doing my father a service by imposing reality on a harmless delusion that he believed, or would I be causing more harm to his confidence and comfort? It was important to ask myself whether I wanted to impose truth and reality on my father for his good, or for my own - for his comfort and well-being, or for mine.

It seemed to me that the best course of action in this regard was to put his needs ahead of my own. I decided that I would encourage him to inhabit whatever reality he wanted, as long as it didn't cause harm to him or anyone else. I encouraged him to tell me whatever thought or story he had in his head at the time and believed to be real. One of us knew what was really going on and how to keep safe, and one is all you need. This was not the limit of my lying, however. The experience of taking over my father's care and affairs was a long, difficult, and exhausting one, largely because he refused to believe he had a problem. Every action or decision became a fight – a negotiation. I had to convince him either to do things himself, or allow me to do things, and then convince him all over again when he forgot our conversations or felt particularly stubborn. I had to list the reasons over and over for a decision, and refute every argument he made against me.

I couldn't force him to do something but I was becoming exhausted by the struggle. Over time, however, I observed that, surprisingly, there were a few tactics my father seemed responsive to – a few things he seemed respectfully afraid of. I learned that there were a few small lies I could use which might get him to do what was necessary. Early on in our journey together, during a conversation about how his care manager needed to be paid so she could keep helping him, my father grew more and more obstructive and paranoid, refusing to believe that he had a problem or anything needed to be done.

My sister and I finally grew so frustrated that she informed him quite firmly that either he agree to sign the payment contract or we were no longer going to be involved in his life at all, would never visit again, and would leave him to (essentially) rot in his own home. I quickly backed her up and even though neither one of us probably could have done it, *he* didn't know that. He believed that we really meant it. Surprisingly, he agreed to sign the contract, whether in fear of our threat, or because some part of him admitted that there really was a problem. I was just happy that the task had been completed and that we had a tool for future encounters, although I knew it was probably something we couldn't use too often. The point is that, because of a harmless untruth, something helpful was achieved and potential harm was averted.

Other times when he was being particularly difficult about losing his driving privileges or having to accept an in-home aide, I explained calmly that it wasn't we his family that wanted all of this, it was "the authorities." My dad appeared to have a healthy respect for the authorities, the police in particular. When I explained that the authorities had gotten my sister and me in trouble the last time he had been found wandering, which was, in fact, true, I added that they had a file on our family and that they required we help him in all these ways or else they would step in and take over. Fortunately, he believed me.

At no time was lying an easy thing to do for me, since I also have a healthy respect for authority and the truth. But I knew at all times that it was for his welfare, and not something I was doing lightly. Stretching the truth a little became an acceptable way to get Dad the care and support that he absolutely needed, regardless of what morality or society thought about it. Perhaps if our situation hadn't been so urgent, we may have come up with more palatable ways to get our father what he needed, but I began to think that since dementia doesn't fight fair, neither should we. How else do you get a paranoid, cognitively-challenged former authority figure to do what you need him to do, and what is in his best interests to do?

Consider this: as adults, there are many truths and topics we would not expose children to. If there is a difficult subject to be discussed, we couch it in terms a child will understand, which will not frighten or disturb them. While I don't advocate treating our care receivers like children, since they are not, I do believe that, like children, their minds and emotional systems are no longer capable of dealing with complex issues, events, and decisions. We must treat our care receivers with the same care and discretion that we do our children. We must be willing to look beyond our past relationship with them and what is comfortable for us. We have to be willing to go against what we've been taught - what is ingrained in us.

Obviously, we aren't advocating lying as a spiritual practice, but I am prepared to acknowledge that there are times when lying is definitely the lesser of two evils. There's no denying that it can really come in handy when you're trying to manage your charge's comfort and well-being. Perhaps it's not what many counselors would agree with, but I firmly believe there are times and instances when not telling the truth is in the best interests of our loved ones, when it is the most appropriate and caring thing to do for them, both in the moment, and in the long term.

As to whether lying leads to loss of dignity and trust by the care-taker, I think that if you continually treat them with dignity and respect, and really feel it, that will come through regardless. In any case, feelings and non-verbal communication have become even more important to a dementia sufferer than words. I ran across this quote, "Meaning is in people, not in the words by themselves." I have to say I really think it says it all.

*

One of the most important tools can also be the hardest to use: taking a break and getting some distance. Don't be afraid to use whatever resources are available to you in terms of respite and relief of your duties. I talk to caregivers who feel guilty for sending their loved one off to respite care because they need a break or are taking a trip. Don't be guilty about using respite care. It gives the disabled or aging individual a social activity and place to go, while providing their caregiver some relief. It is a valuable and vital resource for the family caregiver, allowing them time away from administering care. Caregiving is a stressful, challenging job that takes a physical and emotional toll on caregivers – time off is essential to health and self-care.

Although they can sometimes be a little hard to find, there are federal, state, and community programs for caregivers that offer free or low-cost respite care for family caregivers. Some of the bigger nonprofit organizations also offer subsidized care programs, and there are also adult day care programs available – usually on a sliding cost scale. Some Assisted Living and Extended Care facilities also offer paid respite care; temporary institutional care of an aging or ill individual, providing relief for their permanent caregivers, usually overnight. It provides short to long-term breaks for families or caregivers who might need time for reasons as varied as self-care, a family emergency, or a trip.

Dad attended a weekly day program that I really believe had a positive effect on him. While he was still fairly lucid, he attended a support group for men with dementia, and although I'll never know how much he actually contributed to the discussion, perhaps it helped him to know that other people were experiencing the same things he was. He also created art, gardened, listened to music and had a meal during his visits. Although never a social person, I believe the interaction with the staff and other attendees helped him use his brain and lifted some of the depression he felt. It was a private pay program, partially subsidized by the charity attached to it so low-income families could participate.

Another good reason to investigate respite care is in case of an emergency or other problem. If the primary caregiver cannot work and no family member can provide care, having a place you can trust will respect and care for your loved ones, especially in case of emergency, is vital. Already being familiar with a place you can put your care receiver if necessary is invaluable, as is knowing they are already familiar and comfortable with the facility.

*

In time, you will become this person's whole world - they will take their cues from you and look to you for comfort and guidance. We must be our loved one's guide, prepared to help them deal with scary and unfamiliar situations, new people and environments, and even with the changes happening to their own bodies. Use your whole body as a tool to pick up physical and emotional clues to mood and mental state and to physical and emotional comfort. Be calm and take the time to listen and observe them. They may not be able to alert you verbally to something that they need or want. If they do alert you verbally to something, it may not be in a detailed or coherent way that you can easily understand.

I could usually tell when Dad was feeling depressed or frustrated at what was happening to him because of his face and his actions. He could stiffen up and refuse to move or sit down when I or another caregiver was trying to get him to do something – sometimes he still does. He averts his eyes and his expression becomes even more stony and fixed if he isn't happy. Conversely, when he is feeling good, he may still wink at us, or frown playfully, with one eyebrow up and one down.

I firmly believe that vomiting in Greg's car on the way to the clinic was a visceral, somatic response to something he didn't want to do. Dad doesn't like leaving his home at the best of times and the last few times he had been taken out of it, bad and painful things had happened to him. Since he can no longer speak, all he had left was his body as a way to register his fear and displeasure.

Although I am a physically affectionate person, my father and I did not have a physically affectionate relationship before the dementia. After the dementia, I noticed how well he responded to touches on the arms and back, spontaneous hugs, and pats on the hands. He began to touch me affectionately in ways he hadn't been able to before the dementia. I noticed that I could distract him from something unpleasant by touching his arm and looking him in the eye. I also noticed the comfort I took from his touch.

Often, I could see Dad watching me in an unfamiliar situation for guidance about what he was supposed to do or where he was supposed to go. I found myself cueing him with my body or pointing and suggesting we go a certain way. I never really told him to do anything, I just made suggestions and subtly directed him. There is a saying that 'Invitation always triumphs over insistence', and I think it's really true. In every way, I tried to make him feel that we were in this together, and I think it really helped.

I didn't always know what Dad wanted, or needed, or was really trying to tell me, but I knew he was desperate to be understood. There is a term for this behavior, *perseveration,* which means a tendency for an impression, idea, or feeling to dissipate only slowly and to recur during subsequent experiences due to stimuli or a need to convey an idea of feeling. It causes a care receiver to repeat questions, statements, or behaviors over and over.

It requires awareness, desire, and persistence to make sense of some of the things your charge will try to tell you, and patience to withstand the constant repetition. I found that if I really paid attention to Dad's words, facial expressions, and gestures, I could often figure out what he wanted or was trying to convey. If he was just confused or caught up in an illusion, I just went along with it.

I never got irritated at him or chastised him for repeating himself, although I sometimes felt irritated by it. Dad would tell me the same stories and jokes at least once every half an hour, and each time I acted as if I was fascinated and hadn't heard it before. Sometimes Dad's stories were just an effort to entertain me, sometimes they were a way for him to process what was happening in the present, using his past events and experiences.

His repeated stories about being a flight test engineer seemed like an effort to communicate pride about what he used to do and be. A joke every time we went grocery shopping: "This cart must be Communist because it always pulls to the left!" said with a grin and a mischievous glance, was meant to elicit a laugh from me, and some fellowship. I let myself be silly with him, and be caught up in his world.

At other times, I knew there was something he was trying to convey and the repeating meant he hadn't conveyed it. Asking me repeatedly what time a certain appointment was or whether we had performed a chore that he had determined was vital, was the manifestation of his effort to remain in control or reflected anxiety about what was happening to him. One of Dad's obsessions was wanting to know often where his money was, how much he had, where it was coming from, and how his aides were getting paid. I know that Dad probably felt scarcity all his life but was able to deal with it as a lucid adult. As a cognitively-challenged one, uncertain about what was happening to him and where he would end up, and whether he would be supported, it's not strange that he would obsess about money. I reassured him often about how much money he had.

*

Another reason to really pay attention to your care receiver's behavior is because it can help convey something more serious. We tend to think that worsening behaviors, forgetfulness, and even lassitude and inattention are just because of worsening dementia. They can also represent other problems like infections and pain. Since dementia sufferers can't articulate when something is wrong physically or even emotionally, we must look for other signs.

This has only happened with Dad once, so far, when I didn't realize how much pain he was suffering after his surgery for an infected boil. After I brought him home from the hospital, I noticed that he looked as if he'd been put through a wringer, which wasn't surprising since it was a major intervention. He looked gray and gaunt and exhausted, and he was sitting gingerly on his recliner chair, sort of listing to one side. He was on antibiotics and pain meds, but it was obvious that the boil was still extremely painful. His caregiver, Greg, reported that he seemed quite happy to be back home, however, so I visited with him for a while, then drove to work.

I was surprised and dismayed to get a call from Greg later in the afternoon saying that Dad was sweating and pale and couldn't seem to eat or have a bowel movement. He was worried about another bad infection or something worse, and begged me to take Dad to the ER again. I arranged for Greg to bring him to an ER at a hospital midway between our houses. My husband and I jumped in the car and drove over as fast as evening traffic would permit.

The minute Greg brought Dad in the sliding ER doors, I could see that something was seriously wrong. Like a panicky horse, his eyes rolled in pain and fear and the whites were showing. His legs were stiff and tense, which was making it hard to walk and he was pale, sweating, and clammy - all at once. He was no longer able to speak coherently, but as he stared at me, the appeal to please stop whatever it was that was happening, was clear. He couldn't tell us in words, but his body told us that something serious was going on.

As we stood for a moment in the lobby, Dad started to list to one side and Greg and I had to grab him and hold him upright. I sent Paul off quickly to find a wheelchair, and when we tried to lower Dad into it, he could hardly bend. We neglected to jam a foot behind the chair and the minute we got Dad settled down into it, he almost went over backward, the four of us to grabbing desperately at different parts of the chair in order to keep from depositing him on the floor. Fortunately, the nurse came out quickly to escort us to an exam room.

As I sat next to him in the cubicle, waiting, rubbing his arm and trying to comfort him, I felt helpless. This can be one of the most difficult things about caring for a person with dementia; like children, they lack the ability to tell you exactly what is wrong and where it hurts, and you are forced to waste precious hours trying to determine the problem while they are forced to suffer. And the caregiver has to be the advocate for the care receiver, has to try to translate actions, and behaviors, and garbled words into problems for the medical staff to deal with. I have noticed that doctors and nurses still are not as accustomed to dealing with dementia sufferers as they should be. They kept addressing their questions to my dad until I gently pointed out that he had dementia and couldn't answer their questions coherently. It was up to me to try to give them every fact in an effort to help them solve the problem.

After hearing about the surgery, one of the doctor's first actions, which I heartily applauded, was to give Dad some more pain medication. After an agonizing few hours during which they catheterized Dad to examine his urine and poked and prodded him in various other ways, he began to look much better and less inwardly focused. It was finally determined that the symptoms had been caused because of pain. Greg had not given Dad nearly enough pain meds, relying instead on Tylenol, in part because he disliked overmedicating his residents - something I usually whole-heartedly supported. The poor man had been literally sitting on the hot seat, unable to alert anyone that his suffering had pushed his body too far.

I am *very* pro-pain medication, however, and I felt so badly for my father. After that, I impressed on Greg quite strongly that, while I shared his anti-medication stance, he was to stuff Dad with every pain med he had been given until they ran out. Fortunately, while seriously horrifying and uncomfortable for Dad, it was not something more serious, like a missed bladder or kidney infection. It could have been so much worse, and for others, it has been.

Caregivers have missed signs of serious illness because they just can't tell if agitation and screaming is dementia-related or something else; and have unfairly castigated themselves afterward. Knowing your care receiver well is the best defense against this problem: I am truly fortunate that Dad's caregiver, Greg, is so attuned to him. You won't be able to see or prevent everything, however. We are all human and doing the best job we can. Try to keep an open mind to every possibility. Watch your care receiver for differences in behavior and action. Look for things like not eating, vomiting, anger, agitation, and restlessness.

*

These are the tools of caregiving – feeble and haphazard as they are - a bailing bucket against a tidal wave. These tools are sometimes simultaneously the dilemmas of caregiving: those decisions we must make and actions we must take that are absolutely necessary and appropriate to the health and well-being of ourselves and our care-taker that may also carry negative emotional weight, placed on them by ourselves or others.

Ultimately, you will become your own best caregiving tool. What you see, hear, notice, and feel instinctively and in your gut are all implements in your toolbox. You will know when something is wrong from a change in your care receiver's mood or behavior. You will know that they need support, or comfort, or affirmation. When in doubt, think about what you might need in the same situation, or how you might feel, and go with that. We can never go wrong when we use our empathy and compassion.

I think the central motto of caregiving should be: "Do what is in your care receiver's best interest, and your best interest, according to the dictates and requirements of each moment, without feeling guilty or ashamed." Whether that means lying to your care-taker to keep them from repeatedly feeling the pain of a loved one's death, or placing them in a care facility, or giving them medication that may space them out but will give the both of you relief from difficult behaviors and hallucinations. Do what you have to do without worrying about others' thoughts or expectations and without shaming yourself. Trust your instincts and judgment as a good caregiver, because you are.

A Few Things I Figured Out.

- There are many books detailing valuable coping strategies for dementia and behavior modification techniques. However, the most important strategy or approach to someone with any kind of illness, but especially dementia, is simply to act from your heart and your instinct, with a little common sense thrown in. It is important to have the imagination to put yourself in your charge's place and feel how you would want to be treated and regarded. Be observant, use your instincts, pay attention to gut feelings, don't be afraid to innovate and experiment or be silly with your loved one. These are the tools that all caregivers possess, and can use, and they will be your most effective.

- I believe that people with dementia shouldn't be "kept" in our reality. It is far more comfortable for them, and less agitating, to be allowed to inhabit whatever time and reality they are in during a given moment. I never cared where or when Dad was, and when I toured facilities I made sure their policies on this were the same as mine. Join them in their reality, don't take anything personally, stay calm and positive, show affection and reassurance, and distract or redirect. Often, sticking to an established routine can help. Don't get caught up in whether or not something makes sense to you because it most likely does to your care receiver.

- A person with dementia may not cognitively understand everything but they can still feel things about what is happening. In fact, their distress or anxiety can be amplified when they aren't being understood. You must protect them from any experiential roads down which they can get lost. Don't ask long, complicated questions. Stick to short and sweet and easy to comprehend. Don't ask them to store new information. Interact with them through these past memories, no matter how out of reality they are. Learn from them, always agree, never interrupt or finish a sentence. Let them feel that you are on their side; that the two of you have a "we relationship." There are many excellent books listed in Resources that detail gentle Montessori-like strategies for helping those with dementia.

- Keep in mind that medical personnel are not always well-versed in dealing with dementia. They may continue to address questions to your care receiver that they can't answer. It is up to you to take them aside and make them understand that YOU are the one who has the information and can make the decisions. Make sure you have the proper documentation to support this claim if necessary; a Health Care Power of Attorney, or Living Will, along with the rest of your care receiver's chart.

- I have learned over time that telling untruths, omitting details and withholding information, and affirming incorrect belief systems- all of which might be considered lying-can be some of the most useful and compassionate tools of caregiving. There are times when not imposing the truth on someone is the most compassionate thing you can do for them. It is up to you as the caregiver to decide at what point the truth is still beneficial, and at what point it is time to start lying. Consider, as well, that you can avoid most problems proactively by not bringing up problematic questions or lines of conversation.

- Say what you mean and do what you say you're going to do. Make sure your words, voice, and body language all say the same thing. That is all the truth and respect you need. If it still makes you uncomfortable, try to think about it as lying to the dementia, not to your loved one. Strategies include: finding out what they might respect in terms of the police, social service authorities, or loss of access to you or something else. Please understand that I'm not advocating neglect or abuse used as threats in any way. I'm just not above using any information you have about what will motivate your loved one to act. Your life and your time, as always, are just as valuable. I think, as caregivers, we should be using any and every tool available to us in order to fulfill our roles.

- Use your body. Read between the lines. Keep your eyes watchful, ears tuned in, mind alert, heart open. Follow your instincts and your gut. Those with dementia show their frustration and physical status in different ways. Listen to everything they do and say and everything they don't say. If there are a lot of destructive or acting-out behaviors, consider that it might be the only way sufferers have left of conveying illness or pain, their feelings about what is happening to them, or they are lonely and missing human interaction. For example: urinary tract infections, or any infection in the body, can cause acting-out behaviors. Try to identify and solve the root cause of a problem.

- Respite care can take place in specially-focused facilities, but is also often offered by Assisted Living Facilities or Adult Day Programs. Costs differ, as do hours offered – programs vary in time from part of a day to several days. Programs are usually private pay, however, there are some government programs and subsidies to help with costs. Adult Day programs provide several hours of planned programs, groups, meals, and activities. Finding a place you trust in case of emergency is also vital.

17.

Shift Happens

"'People think it's just forgetting your keys,' she says. 'Or the words for things. But there are the personality changes. The mood swings. The hostility and even violence. Even from the gentlest person in the world. You lose the person you love. And you are left with the shell... And you are expected to go on loving them even when they are no longer there. You are supposed to be loyal. It's not that other people expect it. It's that you expect it of yourself. And you long for it to be over soon.'" Alice LaPlante,

Sometimes I imagine a non-caregiver stumbling on one of our blog posts, or Facebook groups, or an article in USA Today about the burden of caregiving, and asking themselves, "What's the big deal? Yes, it is hard to care for someone else full time, but we do that for our children and we make it through. Parents don't complain this much!" And on the surface, perhaps it does look like we are protesting too much, as Shakespeare would say. However, the most difficult part of caregiving to explain is the emotional toll it takes – not only because we are caring for a loved one who, unlike a baby, won't grow up or get better – but because we are also having to initiate a painful shifts in our entwined roles and personalities.

Giving care to someone with progressive dementia means that you have to give that person up, you have to shift your thinking absolutely, and it's a process that takes time, practice, and awareness. I believe that a lot of the grief and anger surrounding a caregiver and receiver is caused by this refusal to let the emotional structure shift. We don't want our loved ones to change, but the reality is that they already have, and now it is our job as the caregiver to do the same. It involves a shift in your thinking that can be difficult to make.

This person is no longer the person they were, no longer your adult loved one. They haven't just decided to start thinking or acting in a different way – their brain chemistry has changed. In some cases, entire parts of their brain have shut down or atrophied. Dementia works on every part of the brain; erasing information, deleting programs, rewiring communication between systems and organs, shutting down pathways, and inhibiting the cellular chemistry responsible for brain function. Other illnesses can also remove clear thinking and decision-making, and affect memory and behavior. For the most part, none of this stuff is coming back and it can be really hard to take in that the person we knew has changed so fundamentally.

In my experience, the only way for the new relationship between caregiver and care receiver to work smoothly and relatively painlessly is by letting go of who and what your loved one represented for you and dealing with them as an entirely new person. The choice becomes whether to remain trapped in old ideas and patterns, or to focus on learning the new roles in which the situation has placed us, which can lead to personal and emotional growth. Caregiving is about choosing to let go of these patterns that no longer serve us and the ways things used to be in order to meet new needs and events.

*

Caregivers may have a great deal of difficulty making this mental reorganization, at least at first. It is vital that they recognize this person is no longer their husband or wife or parent. It's a crucial

– and incredibly challenging shift in emotions and role. Caregivers need to face up to the fact that the person they knew and loved has shifted. This is a person who doesn't reason in a lucid and intelligent manner anymore. They don't remember dangers and decisions and complex issues. They can't keep themselves safe anymore, and shouldn't be trusted with complex decisions or dangerous tools like cars.

They don't love you or understand you in the same way they once did, and they can't feel the emotions they once felt. They can feel guilt, shame, fear, and regret from *your* reactions to their actions, but they don't self-recognize those feelings like we would. They won't respond to you in the same way, or care for you, or even think about you. They just don't think the same way anymore – the disease has changed them neurologically, systematically, and on a cellular level – and they will never have the facilities they once had. It is essential that caregivers start to see their loved ones clearly and realize they are never coming back as they were but it often only happens after months and months of painful struggle, emotional upset, and confusion.

Wives may detail honestly and practically the progression of their husband's illness, the meds being used, the legal or financial steps being taken, and other practicalities that indicate a total awareness of the presence of the disease. They will then proceed to act and react towards their husband as if they were still of sound mind. They will express anger for certain actions or responses, or get triggered by behaviors, or not understand an impulse or response. They will allow husbands to drive long past the time of safety because they don't want to hurt that husband's pride, or because they need their husband to have capabilities and independence when they no longer do.

Husbands will provide medical details, discuss doctor's visits, behaviors and symptoms, and steps being taken to care for their wives. They will then turn around and be frustrated at an incorrect statement or memory, repeatedly correcting a spouse or berating them for getting it wrong. Or they will let them leave the house alone and unaccompanied after that spouse gets agitated or threatens to leave.

Spouses can have an especially tough time because they want the special emotional structure between themselves and their loved ones not to alter. They may expect a spouse to perform the functions they have always performed, think and act in the ways they have always thought and acted, respond in the ways they have responded – even when the disease has obviously altered that person. It can be difficult to give up the affection, hopes, and dreams invested in that person as a thinking, lucid, capable spouse – even as the evidence of dysfunction and cognitive problems mounts.

Adult children will see that something is wrong with their parent, and may even have persuaded their parent to let them help, but will then let their parent drive long after it is safe. They will hesitate to have difficult financial discussions with their parent because that parent has always been secretive about money. We may become frustrated at their childlike behaviors.

The difficulty inherent in caring for a parent is that we feel strongly that our parents should behave in certain expected ways because that's what we know – that's what we are familiar with. We want our parents to respond the way they have always responded, to look the way they have always looked, and act according to the roles they have played, so that we can then inhabit *our* roles as the children of someone. We may be willing to take on the physical aspects of caregiving for a parent but become angry, or sad when it becomes obvious that the important emotional relationship has shifted without warning. We want that parent back.

*

Emotionally speaking, I didn't really have this problem. My father made my childhood somewhat difficult and we did not have the best relationship as adults. There were a few things about him I was familiar with or accustomed to – ways my heart recognized him as being my father, but there were so many elements about him that were a mystery to me, so many ways in which we were not close or connected, that I felt a peculiar detachment throughout much of his illness. I didn't feel as if I needed to hold on to who he was which made it almost easy to adjust to who he became in his illness – the new person I would meet each day. I accepted each person that showed up.

Sometimes he joked and laughed with me and was silly, teasing me about the coins scattered on the floor of my car. Other times, he was depressed and withdrawn, a personality I knew well from his depression in my childhood; the difference was that I could see his vulnerability this time, his fear about what was happening to him, and I was grown up and secure enough to make an effort to break through it and get him talking. Perhaps it made it easier to deal with his dementia because he *wasn't* the best Father - we weren't terribly close and there didn't turn out to be much that I missed about him, like I missed about my mom. I never wanted him "back", or wished that he was the Dad he used to be. You can't have back what you never had to begin with. Perhaps if your relationship with your loved one was similar to ours, you'll understand.

For those people who are unlike me – who are closer to their loved ones and know more intimately everything they think and feel and have experienced – those people may have a harder time as the disease progresses. They may have difficulty adjusting to the loss of all they have known, valued, recognized, and depended on and they may fear that they will have difficulties forging connections to who that person is now. While it may make it more difficult and heart-breaking that this person is changing, you are fortunate to have had that closeness, those bonds. You won't lose them, they will just change.

When I think about being a young person and watching my aunt take care of my grandmother, the one thing that stands out was my aunt's insistence on reminding my grandmother who and where she was; contradicting her stories and correcting her when she called someone by the wrong name. At the time, I couldn't understand the harm in just letting my grandmother think or believe whatever she wanted, whether or not it was correct. As I think about it now, however, after having actually been a caregiver, I realized why it might have been so important for my aunt to keep her in the here and now: She still wanted to be the daughter of a mother who was present in the world. My aunt was prepared to care for my grandmother physically, but I suspect she worked hard to keep my grandmother mentally in the present because she wasn't ready to accept any changes - she wasn't yet ready to let go of her mother, or of being a daughter.

Unfortunately, we don't receive a dementia manual at the time of diagnosis. People may sit us down and tell us that the person we have always known will change and is disappearing, but there isn't as much discussion about how the emotional structures we have always known will shift. This is where support groups and talking to other caregivers comes in handy. Find out how everyone else is doing it. It's natural to want the people you love and depend on remain as they are; natural, but not always possible or realistic. You must become someone new, as well, as you take a different role for your loved one.

*

In practical terms, caregiving is about being in control of another human – keeping them safe and doing what is in their best interest. Caring for someone with dementia means stepping in to make decisions and be responsible for someone who has done that for themselves. It means caring for a person who will henceforth need everything done for them while weathering that person's inevitable and understandable anger and resentment, usually focused on you. It means caring for their physical needs to a bigger and bigger degree. It can also mean helping that person come to terms with the emotional issues surrounding their illness. It means being a parent, in the best possible sense of that word.

I think most of us would know instinctively what needs to happen to keep a child safe – how to act and react with someone small, unformed, and unsophisticated who needs your care and is used to being directed. Caring for a parent has an extra sort of difficulty in that this person is *not* a child. This is someone who is accustomed to being an independent adult. Telling a parent that they can no longer drive, for example, because you say so, will not be taken well. Trying to take over finances may spark anger and resentment. This person once had some sort of authority and maturity over you. You may both find it had to forget that. This is where I had most of *my* issues with the shift.

When I took Dad and his life on I couldn't find a lot of information about parenting a parent. Few effective strategies, no suggested phrasing, no plans of action. I had to learn as I went and deal with the questions as they came up. How do you take over the life of an independent, although no longer functioning, adult who has been your authority figure? And how do you force your own parent to do the things you know are best for them, when they refuse to do anything? How do you flip the energy of a relationship so that power that flowed in one direction now flows in another? How do I trump my own Father, who, let's face it, was clinging to his authority and superiority with every last fingernail?

First of all, as caregivers in charge, you are stepping out of a traditional role and taking over your parent's life, which can be confusing since you are no longer deferring to your parent or soliciting their participation or guidance. You may depend on the relationship the way it currently is as a way of navigating your own life, in which case you must decide what you will do when you no longer have the authority figure against which to measure yourself. Most children strive endlessly to earn the approval of their parents, fueling a rise to great heights, or causing despair and failure. Once you reach a certain age, it tends to get a little easier as you become practiced at running your own life and making, and living with, your own decisions. Generally, though, a parent's influence is still there giving you something to either aspire to or something to agitate against, like an oyster and a grain of sand. A little part of me had always had Dad's influence to fight against, which sometimes resulted in a pearl, sometimes not.

As all adult children must do, I had struggled against his belief systems and opinions in an effort to develop my own, and yet I still felt the shadow strings of Dad and his opinions and beliefs, as these had become what I measured myself against. As a daughter, I had always sought his love and approval and feared his poor opinion of me, while at the same time wanting to do things the way I wanted to. Caring for Dad helped me to see that he was not the giant I had made him out to be. Like us all, he could be deeply flawed in both actions and beliefs. He could no longer punish me with silence or disapproval or crushing opinion. I was on my own in life.

The second difficult, yet necessary, thing was to break out of the power roles we inhabited as Father and Daughter. At first I found it incredibly hard to make decisions, stand up to him, and tell him how things were going to be without feeling like he was going to judge me or balk at my direction, which he did anyway. It was also a constant struggle to get through both his ingrained desire for privacy and his dementia-induced paranoia in order to make sense of his affairs. I was trying to establish a position of authority over someone who had always been independent and in charge of their own life and who was paranoid of others' interference.

I was not used to being in control, and was unused to making important decisions without second-guessing myself with questions of what Dad would do or expect or want. There were several other instances, mostly to do with money, when he attempted to maintain control of the situation, and I finally had to start thinking in a different way. One afternoon, Dad was helping me pay bills since he could still write and sign checks and I wanted him to feel useful. He disliked seeing check after check go out, representing money being spent, and he started fighting me with each and every check I asked him to write. I persevered patiently until he lost his temper and threw a signed check at me, at which point, I decided the bad behavior had gone on long enough.

Surprising the both of us, I told him sternly that the bills were his, not mine, for services provided to him, and that I was helping him. I told him if he continued to act rudely, I would leave and not help him anymore, which had the effect of calming him down and apologizing. As my therapist pointed out, he's allowed to be angry but he's not allowed to bite the hand that feeds him.

As I practiced making decisions and assuming authority and directing him, I found it got easier and more natural, until I realized I was confident in my abilities and my position. I had the authority to begin performing important tasks without him and the benefits were numerous. Taking him out of the equation allowed him to think about things that were less stressful than money and what cognitive functions he was losing, and once I wasn't spending precious time and energy negotiating around him, I could get more done and be less angry at him. There were times, though, as I was making big decisions for him that I had to deal with the feeling that I was doing something he would never do, or never approve of. When I eventually sold his house, I was so afraid. I worried whether I was doing the right thing and whether he would approve. It was a unique and valuable piece of property that my family had owned for forty years and I worried that I was selling it in the wrong way, for the wrong amount, to the wrong people – and that Dad would come to life somehow and be furious.

The knowledge that what you are doing may adversely affect your care receiver must be faced each time you make a decision. I'm quite certain that Dad found it just as difficult to cede control as it was for me to assume it, although he didn't talk about it. I could tell by his attitude and actions, however, that this was not what he wanted. Having someone else taking charge and making decisions for him must have been excruciating.

Taking away control over the trappings of independence like money and transportation is a tough thing for both care giver and care receiver. There are so many questions. How do wives who always cared for husbands allow themselves to be cared for? How do you avoid stomping all over each other's boundaries and hurting each other's feelings? If your husband has been accustomed to paying the bills and managing the money, it will be difficult to take that from him. If you are used to him performing that task, it may be hard for *you* to take it on. Dad's cognition fluctuated over the years until he no longer seemed to want autonomy – only comfort and companionship – so there is a light at the end of the tunnel. Your care receiver will hopefully forget about certain things, and may have different priorities and interests. They will definitely become more dependent on you. Eventually, the only emotional reaction you will have to deal with is your own, since you are still aware of the hardships of parenting an adult.

*

It can be hard to see an adult – especially a parent - *not* act like an adult by behaving poorly or unexpectedly. Or as my friend put it, "When you have a two year old, a thirteen year old, and a Senior Citizen in one body – sitting in your living room, pouting." It can also be incredibly frustrating. Parents are our roots, our foundation. To see our parents as vulnerable or different is hard; we don't want to see any flaws or failings, nor do we want to see them get weaker in any way, or act differently from how they've always acted. I occasionally had trouble with this.

Dad exhibited most of the recognizable dementia behaviors; stubbornness, forgetfulness, repetition of phrases and requests, annoying and sometimes destructive actions, and mood swings. I often found myself becoming triggered emotionally by how he was acting and the ways he was changing. There were times when I felt intense feelings of anger and impatience, whether it was because he wouldn't do what I was asking him to, or was repeating a question or phrase so many times it would drive me crazy, or because he was doing something inappropriate out in public.

When I would bring this anger and frustration to my therapist, she would point out that a professional caregiver with no ties to my father would see him as a patient, and regard these behavioral issues as regular and expected. It would most likely not trigger him or her if my father repeated a statement over and over again, or became childishly moody and refused his dinner; they would expect it to happen and most likely deal with it calmly and compassionately. *I*, however, was reacting to him as my father, bringing to the incident all the emotional stories from the past, and allowing it to trigger me into anger.

The situation required a delicate balancing act between love and compassion for my father and the detachment of a caregiver, and, with assistance, I became better at walking that line. Your response to your caregiver must be careful and mindful and you must allow that shift in thinking to happen. But you must also be gentle with yourself and allow yourself to make mistakes and regress into old ways of thinking. It can be hard to avoid getting triggered by your loved one's refusal to cooperate or their interesting new personal and behavioral habits. And it can be hard to deal with their grief and rage at this process; be aware that you may have trouble helping them with their feelings.

*

One of the things I had the most difficulty with was helping my dad with his feelings about what was happening. It is not easy to help a care receiver with the emotions caused by the losses they are suffering, while avoiding being triggered by the behaviors and emotions they are exhibiting. It's important to be aware that your loved ones will be grieving and enraged and disappointed and resentful about the ways that age and illness are destroying their lives. I am sure that some of Dad's attitudes and stubbornness and bad behavior were motivated by his frustration and grief at the loss of control, not only over his life and decisions, but also over his body. His mind was betraying him, and his entire life was turning upside down - he must have been feeling terrible grief, anger, and confusion. Having to give up control of his car and his finances were two of the hardest things he had to do. Accepting the presence of in-home aide was also incredibly difficult, and he was angry and upset about it for weeks.

I was able to recognize that he was struggling and I tried to be as empathetic and compassionate as possible, but there were some things I just found I couldn't help him with. There were times when I complained to my therapist about the impossibility of helping him deal with his feelings, specifically because he was my father, and in general because I was grieving and angry, too. I didn't feel capable of acting the therapist to my father, and there were limits to how well I could guide him emotionally through this terrible situation.

A spouse caregiver may experience this a little differently. It may be easier to help in this way because of the marriage's history of helping each other deal with and work through difficult issues. Again, however, this person represented a particular role - with strengths and capabilities - that they no longer have, which may be challenging to accept with equanimity. Be aware of lashing out at your care receiver for not being able to soothe or manage their own emotions and make sure you have someone to listen to *your* feelings and problems in the ways your spouse did for you.

*

It can be so difficult to make the type of emotional shift caregiving requires of us: in essence, to continue to love this person while knowing they are not the person you originally loved. It requires loving them in a whole new way, and it can be a tough adjustment to make. Making the adjustment as soon as possible will save you heartache and stress in the long run, however, and it will make things easier for your care receiver. Keep your memories of the person they used to be strong, and look clearly at the person now in front of you.

It can also be difficult not to be impatient with the changes we are seeing in our care receivers, and the struggles they may be making against these changes – and against us as the controllers of their lives. Try to remember how angry, afraid, and sad it made you feel when you were young or in a situation you were powerless to affect. Letting go of the fear attached to inevitable role change allowed me more peace, and the ability to truly believe that I was acting in the best interest of my loved one. The truth is that it never stops being a difficult process and each family is going to follow its own path. There are days when the changes are easier to accept and days when they are not. Some individuals have less positive results, some more positive, some people are able to put the past behind them, and some are not; there are no perfect results.

This is an entirely new person, who in many ways resembles your loved one, but is not the same person. Trying to deal with them as if they were the person they used to be is no longer possible. It is possible, however, to still care for this person in just the same way, with respect and understanding. You can still love this person. My hope for you is that you find that there are rewards in this new relationship that you couldn't have foreseen.

A Few Things I Figured Out.

- If you are fighting against the realities of the situation - that your loved one is ill and changing by the minute from the person you knew and loved into someone you don't - it is going to cause nothing but suffering and turmoil. Continuing to act and react towards them in accustomed ways won't work. It is good to remember them as they were, but continuing to deal with them as if they were still the person you knew will not help the situation. By necessity, roles will change. If necessary, find inconspicuous ways to provide assistance and allow your loved ones to save face whenever possible. Make choices according to what you feel is in their best interests and health. Their privacy is, of course, important, but their safety must be paramount. It can be incredibly hard for a parent to accept dependence on anyone, let alone their child, who used to be in the dependent role. It can be difficult to give up the dependence you may have had on your spouse for certain things, and difficult for them to give up what they are used to doing.

- Responding with love and caring is always appropriate, regardless of the actions or reactions of your charge. Living with what is and accepting your new world and loved one as they are can reduce suffering and make space for new possibilities and emotions. You can still have a relationship with your care receiver – it will just look differently from how you expected. Consider that you may be interacting with a new person, someone who is open in different ways or thinks and feels in different ways than they used to. Consider as well that this person may change each and every day, moving further away from what you knew about them and what they represented for you. Grieve this loss. However, you may like the new person who emerges – I did! Dad and I developed a whole new, affectionate relationship.

- You can't plan for every event and encounter and emotion. Like all good parenting, caregiving is about facing issues, not avoiding them. There is no good time to do the hard stuff, no perfect day or way to switch roles. At some point, you will be the bad guy. Sooner or later you will do to your spouse or your parents what your parents did to you when you were little - make decisions you didn't like and didn't understand that were geared towards your care and safety. At best, you can try to keep yourself centered, feel what you're feeling, be respectful and fall apart later. Then do it again the next day.

- It is possible that others may also have difficulty seeing or accepting that your roles have changed. Other family members, who may be in denial or are unversed with the entire situation, may have difficulty. They may criticize how you are speaking to your loved one, or that you are doing things for them. They may try to undermine your authority.

- I didn't expect to be so triggered by Dad's emotions, behaviors, and attitudes. Caregiving blurs boundaries and makes things just that much more difficult; try to keep yours clear. Decide what you are capable of doing that doesn't cross firm boundaries and ask, or pay, for help with those that do. Decide what behaviors you are willing to put up with. When you are dealing with an almost complete personality and behavior change from the person you knew, try to remember that you are dealing with negative aspects of the disease, not the person you love - it is the disease that is causing the bad behavior. You have to look beyond any feelings of disrespect or anger you may be experiencing as a result of the swap in roles and power, it does get easier. Remember who they were and why they might be feeling this way and it will help you to be compassionate and respectful. Keep appropriate boundaries - they are not allowed to bite the hand that feeds them, bad behavior is never allowed. Be patient, but be firm, and take no abuse.

- Your loved ones will be having their own difficult feelings about the situation. I'm not sure why I didn't realize this would happen, and when it did I wasn't sure whether I had the ability or the desire to help my father navigate through this experience. I think participating in his Men's Group was helpful, but in many ways, he went through a lot of emotional hardship on his own. There's no shame in asking for help from a professional if you can't. Be aware also that you can be influenced by their emotions. You can take steps to help your loved one deal with them, without taking them on as your own. Remember that they will be struggling with the same fear, grief, and anger that you are.

18.

There Are Apps for This!?!

"Any sufficiently advanced technology is indistinguishable from magic." Arthur C. Clarke

Speaking of tools, one of the main things that caregivers have going for us now is technology. The creation and growth of the Internet has changed the nature of healthcare, illness, information gathering, community, and caregiving immensely. The web has become a lifeline for caregivers in that it allows for better access to more information and resources: resources that never used to be in such a centralized location. When I started caregiving, we didn't have this incredibly useful tool.

I am a child of the seventies and eighties and as such, I am in that generational limbo between being comfortable with computers and knowing almost nothing about them. About half of my generation went towards the emerging technologies early and have followed it to where it is now. The other half, me included, didn't, and have kind of played catch up to achieve even the modicum of tech knowledge that we have. Those generations before me are largely in that same boat: if they are interested in learning how to use computers, they seek that knowledge out, if not, they don't. Generations *after* me have the enviable facility with technology born of growing up with it.

Whichever camp you come from, some sort of computer knowledge is becoming essential and the use of technology in all walks of life will only increase and expand. I have been witness to this growing expansion (I remember when there were no cell phones or ATMs) as it affected life in general but what I have found most interesting in the ten years I have been giving care is how technology has changed the ability of caregivers to give care and survive. Technology, specifically the Internet, has changed the experience that is caregiving for the better, and thank God, because something had to!

I started caregiving in 2003, when Facebook was still just on college campuses and something called a "weblog" had only taken off a few years prior. Google as a presence was only about four years old. We had Yahoo and email, of course, and AOL, and something called Netscape, and I had started to be able to access information and entertainment on-line. If I'd been more tech-aware, I probably would have been able to find important and helpful stuff even then, but I muddled along as best as I could. I, and most other caregivers, still looked for information about dementia and caregiving in the Yellow Pages, in books, and through contact with big organizations like the Alzheimer's Association.

The first time I looked for a facility to move Dad into, in 2006, I was given a large packet of documents binder-clipped together by Dad's care manager, Kathryn. The packet listed most of the facilities in King County as well as their specifics; directors, number of apartments, health department results, amenities, etc. I laboriously went through the pile manually with a pen, making phone calls and arranging visits with the ones I liked, crossing off the ones I didn't. The only way to see the facilities was to visit them in person.

As time went on, of course, I began to use the Web to find more and more information, entertainment, and connection to others, but it took me a while to realize just how much the Web was starting to change my caregiving experience. One of the first signs was the establishment of my blog, in 2009, and I thought that was pretty daring. I started using the Internet to look up other blogs and forums and from there I discovered the Lewy Body Dementia Association's website, as well as the site of the Alzheimer's Association and many more. As I found more good websites, I linked to them on my blog. It became a matter of course to search for the information I needed on-line.

When it was time to move Dad again, in 2010, there was no huge packet of printed-out facility information. Large facilities, as well as facility and in-home care search services had gone cyber: all their information was spread out on my computer screen in full color – sometimes with 3-D tours! I then realized just how often I was providing on-line resources to the caregivers I was talking to. Books have always been my preferred source for information, and there are a few books I always recommend to people, but websites and forums had begun to make up the bulk of my referrals. I recommended informational links and search engines to caregivers, as well as on-line support forums. The Web was also becoming the main source of information for my own research and writing.

It wasn't until I was doing research for this book that I really realized how far technology for caregiving had advanced because I found out there are actual apps for caregiving! I should have known considering there seems to be an app for everything else, although admittedly, this is an aspect of phone and computer technology I don't really have a handle on. I Googled caregiving apps and found some that performed tasks like storing and emailing personal health records, tracking and organizing caregiver tasks, managing medications and possible drug interactions, and tracking things like vital signs.

Ten years has made a huge difference in what technology can offer those who give care. I am not the most tech-savvy person compared to other people I know, and I certainly don't use my smart phone and my laptop now as the tools for a new age as much as I could. I don't really tend to stretch my technology wings very often, however, even I have fully turned to the Web.

*

Like a mini-library, the Internet contains lists of local and national government resources and how to obtain them. There is a great deal of information about types of care, including sites like, *A Place for Mom,* a database that connects caregivers and families with care resources and professional caregivers. There are multiple sites that list different types of care facilities, including locations, amenities, and performance histories. Most clinics, doctors, and hospitals now have web presences and often some helpful general information. And, of course, sites like the Lewy Body Dementia Association are easy-to-access clearing houses of information on everything from healthcare to housing.

The availability of general health information has become invaluable. Individuals can now research symptoms, illnesses, treatment options, and medications on-line, instead of relying solely on doctors to decide what they are suffering from and what kind of care they can have. We have the opportunity to take charge of our own health and healthcare, and people are doing exactly that, researching problems and solutions in ways that would have been difficult or impossible in the past.

Less well-known syndromes are getting their own cyber faces – helping the public and health care professionals to determine what a disease might be and how to treat it. Alzheimer's is the most common, and commonly diagnosed, type of dementia but for years, people have struggled with loved ones whose symptoms and behaviors didn't fit with Alzheimer's. Looking up symptoms on-line has been one of the main ways that people caring for those with Lewy body and frontotemporal dementias have been able to find support, information, and possibly a new diagnosis, as well as doctors specializing in each particular disease.

There is a caveat to all of this medical knowledge being freely and easily available. We should definitely be cautious when it comes to looking up symptoms and medications. We all know we've become medical experts through the Internet. My friends and I have self-diagnosed ourselves with everything from brain tumors to Braxton-Hicks contractions, so one has to be careful. We should always consult a medical professional if there is a question of serious illness.

*

The Internet can also help caregivers do the practical things they need to do, quickly and easily. Ordering groceries, medical supplies, and pharmaceuticals on-line has become a painless way to have everything a caregiver needs delivered right to their door. I discovered on-line banking for Dad's account, which has been a huge time and energy saver. I have certain bills set up to be paid automatically each month, and can quickly go on-line and pay other random bills. I love not having to make the time to write out checks.

There are so many new products available for a care receiver's comfort, amusement, health and safety that are available on-line. Special clothing, activities and videos, home safety items, and services such as electronic location if a patient wanders. Having such a breadth of services, products, entertainment, and supplies available at the touch of a button and the click of a link is a huge blessing for those who have limited time and energy.

We can also install high-tech, tiny cameras in our homes or the homes of our care receiver and use our Smart phones to monitor their activities and well-being when we are not at home. We can be alerted to a problem or fall just by being able to view them remotely. There are also so-called, "nanny cams," cameras hidden inside household objects that can help us monitor how people are treating our care receiver in our absence.

Unfortunately, the rise in Internet use has also led to new scams and ways for the elderly and infirm to be taken advantage of. Dangerous investment schemes, bogus email requests, fake cures and medications, and too-good-to-be-true offers can be hard to resist and can cause physical and financial damage. Make sure you and your care receiver are aware of and protected from pitfalls like these. Don't give out personal information unless you are sure of who you are providing it to. Don't order from websites that don't have security systems in place.

Perhaps most importantly, the growth of the Internet has allowed caregivers, care receivers, friends, and family members to find community. In fact, this may be what helps us most to deal with new demands in a new age. We can now exchange information and support in ways not possible before. Every day, thousands of people find help, support, and valuable resources; share information and personal stories; and connect to the huge network of caregivers in this country and others. It is to our benefit that we have more forums and outlets than ever to share our experiences and information, and more places to get the information and resources we are going to need to succeed.

Blogs, forums, and Facebook groups have become the new support group. We are able to learn more about what is happening now, what might be coming, and new and better coping mechanisms through reading about other's experiences. The Internet has created an extended network of people dealing with the same issues and struggles, and made it possible for those who cannot leave their homes or who live in isolated areas to reach out and find support. While I still think in-person support groups provide an unmatched support experience, on-line groups can still provide a great deal of help if a care giver is unable to get to one in person or there isn't one in their area.

Because of the wonderful rise in self-publishing and the availability of the Internet for blogging and websites, accounts by caregivers sharing the personal details, problems, and discoveries of their experiences are becoming more common - each one so individual yet so important, that a reader can come away from each with something different. I read a lot of these books and blogs, and though everyone's experiences and focus are different, with different details, the same themes keep popping up - the same foundations to the stories - like the warp and weft threads in a weaving.

It is a testament to the nature of caregivers that these courageous souls are telling their stories, not only in an effort to understand their situation, but also to help others. Everyone wants and needs to tell their stories. Most caregivers I talk to have to go into immense detail, from the very first symptom to what is happening currently, before they can go on to their specific question or issues. All of these accounts are necessary, because they are helping to complete a mosaic of a human experience that is as old as humanity. Everyone should be able to find a story that is similar to their own.

If you're just starting out as a caregiver now, you are lucky, in a way, because those before you did not have this wealth of information and support at their fingertips. Phone apps for caregiving are only the newest in what will hopefully be a lot of new technological aides and advances. As a caregiver advocate, I am so happy to have more information than ever before to offer to those I help and I am looking forward to seeing what is next.

As with all amazing and powerful inventions, the Internet has its drawbacks and dangers, its weaknesses and negatives, and should be handled cautiously. However, I firmly believe it is one of our strongest weapons against the challenges, downfalls, and difficulties of caregiving and living with illness.

A Few Things I Figured Out.

- The Internet had barely gotten started when I began caregiving, but now the amount of information and support is astounding. It has become a crucial and important resource – use it! Forums, blogs, media outlets, Facebook groups, on-line videos, on-line groups, Twitter, and websites like the LBDA and Family Caregiving Alliance are just a few of the many places to find help.

- Let your DSL connection and Smartphone become the indispensable tools they are. Download apps and other helpful programs. Search out websites and links that list vital information and resources. There are more on-line organizations than ever before to support caregivers, including the LBDA, the Alzheimer's Foundation, Caregiver.com, and others. More local governments, health organizations, hospitals, and hospices are going on-line and listing valuable tools and information in easy to find ways.

- You can install cameras in your loved one's house, if they choose not to move to a facility, and use your Smartphone to allow you to monitor those cameras as well as other house systems to keep your care receiver safe.

- Find a forum or forums that you like and sign up. There are great Facebook groups aimed at those who have illnesses as well as their caregivers. Facebook's Memory People, for example, is a closed group for those suffering from dementia and also for caregivers of the disease, but it is not hard to get into. It provides a forum for those affected by dementia to talk about their lives. In the early stages of their illness, set your care receiver up on one of these groups so they have an outlet for what they are experiencing. Don't forget to set yourself up, too. Find blogs that you like to read and make comments – it can be a great way to meet other caregivers. Most of the big sites like the LBDA and Alzheimer's Association have forums but there are many smaller caregiver support sites that have them, as well. Find one you like.

- Create a blog for yourself as a way to journal about your experiences and share with others. Even if nobody else reads it, writing about problems and challenges is a great way to process them.

- Start a blog or Facebook page on behalf of your care receiver. Post photos, health updates, progress, and other information. This can be a great place for others to go to find out how your care receiver is doing. Provide the web address to family and friends instead of you spending valuable time and energy keeping everyone updated. People can also comment, send messages, donate money, and show their support. Many relatives start blogs and FB pages after their loved one's death as a memorial and place to share information.

19.

Chronic Caregiving.

"The number one root of all illness, as we know, is stress." Marianne Williamson

I have now suffered from rheumatoid arthritis (RA) and its attendant difficulties for over half my life. It has had an effect on every area of my adult life, influencing and affecting my appearance, my abilities, my dreams, my level of activity, and my self-worth. At times, my illness has made itself known quite loudly, through painful and debilitating flare ups that left me bed-bound for weeks or months. For the most part, however, it has crept slowly and quietly through my joints, muscles, and tissues, causing low-level inflammation, constant pain, joint deformities, and perpetual fatigue.

Over time, my illness has attempted to crumple me up like a discarded piece of paper; shortening tendons and tissues, atrophying muscles, and drawing my joints up into severe flexion. I have spent many years fighting this concerted effort by my body – using tools like exercise, stretching, Pilates, massage, and Rolfing to keep myself relatively straight and functioning.

Rheumatoid lives with me always – it is a constant dialogue, a perpetual accompanist. For twenty-two years, it has been a factor in my professional choices, my personal and relationship choices, and my care of Dad - both emotionally and physically. It was critical in my choice to care for him at all, and it has influenced the type of care I have provided to him. Every event in my life, from making a meal, to moving, to marrying has been affected by my illness, and it has not remained static in its effects, symptoms, or manifestations.

When I entered my forties a few years ago, a time that can initiate the beginning of the physical challenges of aging for everyone, I noticed a distinct system-wide slowing down. There is a natural wear and tear exerted on the body by forty years of life - I suspect most people in their forties begin to feel new and unwelcome physical ailments and restrictions around this time. I was not immune to those changes, and they were exacerbated by the fact that I have the physicality of a sixty-year-old, not a forty-year-old. I hadn't ever imagined what would happen when those years began to weigh on me and was surprised at their growing impact. I could feel how much harder it was getting to keep myself going.

I had also just gotten married to a man I met two years before, and we were going through all the transitions and growing pains that occur when two people join their lives. The year leading up to the wedding had been exciting and full of planning and events, the wedding itself, which took place on Kauai in October, had been beautiful and fun. However, it was now over, and we were settling in to married life, winter was coming, and I found myself feeling incredibly worn out and fatigued.

I was just not bouncing back, mentally or physically, from my daily struggles like I was accustomed to. My get up and go was evidently already gone. I realized that it was possible that, along with the emotional and physical let-down after my exciting year, I was also experiencing a minor flare up, which was causing some of the extra pain, stiffness, and fatigue. I felt like I was dragging myself around, unable to perform daily chores and errands, let alone the little activities that made me happy.

Just when the small flare up started to improve due to a new medication that my rheumatologist gave me, I started to notice problems I suspected were related to my *pain* medication. For years, I've been on strong pain medication to help combat the almost constant pain from the structural damage and inflammation caused by the Rheumatoid arthritis. I don't really like having to take these meds. In fact, sometimes they feel like a leash that I am tethered to; a leash that lets me move and gives me room and a certain amount of freedom but which is firmly anchored in regular doctor visits and regular applications of medication.

I researched my symptoms on the Internet and discovered I might be feeling the same physical effects that people in withdrawal do! I immediately went to my pain doctor and described the problem, and he agreed with me that my body was developing a tolerance to the medication. He proposed a new non-opioid pain medication that he thought would work well for me. The only problem was that I had to get all the other drugs out of my system before I could try it. I had to go through detox.

You probably won't be surprised to learn that detox is very unpleasant. Every day I felt more tired and I was in a little more pain. I still had a little bit of the old medication in my system when I started the new one, which was not recommended but I was miserable, so I put the new patch on and hoped for the best. What followed was an entire weekend of pain, stiffness, discomfort, dizziness, fatigue, headaches, and stomach pain so bad I couldn't sleep for two days.

The new drugs finally kicked in and they seemed to be working just fine on the pain and fatigue; not quite as well, perhaps, as the old medications but well enough. I continue along my path now, hoping never to have to do something similar again. But this is what it is like to have a chronic illness. Just when you think the earth is firm beneath your feet, it crumbles – sometimes a little, sometimes quite a lot. It is a constant juxtaposition of negotiation and refusal, compromise and stubbornness, hope and hopelessness, rage and acceptance, feeling well and feeling crappy. As anyone knows who has ever had a serious chronic illness, it takes over – if not all of your life, then at least a major part of it. As much as you will let it, sometimes. It becomes a job, a family member, a constant presence to be considered when considering anything about your life.

*

It used to be that I was the only person I knew with a chronic illness but over time that has changed and I have met a disturbingly high number of people who suffer from similar illnesses and problems. 125 million Americans currently suffer with a chronic illness – and by the year 2020, that number is expected to rise to 157 million. Currently, among the working-age population, 45 per cent have a chronic condition. To illustrate just how staggering that is, the numbers equal nearly one in two Americans who suffer from a chronic condition.

People are working, raising children, going to school, and living their lives, while also carrying the burden of a chronic illness.

Just trying to have any kind of normal life while dealing with a long-term illness is a huge challenge – which I can attest to! It can be like having an extra job or family member that you have to take care of. Imagine living your life and doing everything you do while constantly carrying around a huge anchor that you can't put down.

Well people don't understand the extra financial, emotional, and energetic burden of an illness: the time and money spent on getting medical care and having to pay for expensive medications; dealing with medication changes and side effects; keeping a normal job in the face of pain, fatigue, and large numbers of sick days; the demands of relationships, including spouses and children; trying to perform all the daily chores and errands of living while feeling sick. The list goes on.

Unfortunately, people with chronic illnesses aren't exempt from the unlucky odds of caregiving; they are just as likely as anyone else to have a caregiving situation arise in their family. However, if you do already suffer from a chronic illness, you are going into the boxing ring of caregiving with one hand tied behind your back. You already have a person to take care of – yourself! And you may already be lacking the energy and abilities that giving care absolutely demands.

Anyone suffering from a chronic illness knows that there is usually excessive fatigue that comes along with the disease. Fatigue is hard for the medical community to quantify but it can be devastating on the abilities and energy needed to live one's life and care for oneself – let alone caring for another. Fatigue, to me, feels like someone constantly pressing down on my shoulders, weighing me down and restricting what I am able, and desiring, to do.

Chronic illness also often comes with pain, or joint and muscle dysfunction. It may include vertigo or nausea, or an inability to think clearly. It may involve insomnia or an inability to sleep comfortably. It may require dependence on harsh medication, with difficult side effects. It may also include depression and/or other mental issues. Depression is 15-20% higher for the chronically ill than for the average person. All of these will make caregiving more of a challenge

Statistically speaking, since almost a third of our population is caring for an ill or disabled relative, it is inevitable that caregiving and chronic illness will collide. And, in fact, three-fifths of people who are already caregivers aged 19-64 reported fair or poor health and one or more chronic conditions. There is no getting around the fact that being a caregiver when you have a chronic illness is going to be tough.

Dad's dementia has been progressing for at least thirteen years now and I have had to pace myself throughout. When I decided to take on his care, I was concerned about how it would be to essentially have two diseases in my life, and whether it would adversely affect my own condition. Over-stimulation and physical and emotional stress - all of which I expected to experience - are things that can potentially bring on a flare up of my disease so I was wary of how much I would be asked to do.

*

My father was very fit and one of the only things that calmed him down mentally was physical exercise, and he needed constant supervision while he did it. I also knew that I couldn't chase after him if he suddenly decided to take off, which had happened. I just wasn't as strong or as fit as he was, and I wouldn't be able to cope with him physically if something happened. I just wasn't sure I was up to the task. I also suspected that the emotional stresses of our complicated situation and past relationship might exacerbate my condition, which has an emotional component.

Just to be spending a lot of time with my father would have been difficult under normal circumstances. The fact that the man who had neglected to care for many of my needs throughout my life, now needed my care for *his* needs was a difficult one to swallow. I knew I would be filled with resentment if caring for *him* made *me* sicker. I did not want to be a martyr to this particular cause. Luckily, with the help of my therapist and my friends, I have mostly been able to manage, although there have been problems and changes.

When I lived with him, I did suffer from extra fatigue, and from sore joints and muscles when I did too much or walked too far while we were together. Several times I rented a wheel chair and had him push me along some of our favorite walkways. However, the added stress of caring for my father, as well as the extra energy output required, definitely contributed to changes in my disease and wear and tear on my body.

In my mid-thirties, my doctor determined that, apparently not content with just one autoimmune disorder, my body had decided to include another – Fibromyalgia. Fibromyalgia is still not a well-understood condition, but it is thought to be caused by over-active nerves responding to unknown stimuli and it can cause fatigue and serious muscle and tissue pain, with no evident cause. It is a disease suffered most commonly by women, and, unfortunately, until recently, many doctors dismissed women's complaints of pain and fatigue as, "being in your head."

Fortunately, it is now being taken more seriously and more medications are being developed to address it. A change in my medication helped alleviate the symptoms, but it is also something I will deal with the rest of my life. For the most part, I have been able to respect my physical limitations, work through many emotional issues, enjoy caring for and living with Dad, and continue to have my own life, without having a serious flare-up of my condition.

Many caregivers aren't this lucky, either because they have to work too hard in giving care, or because the added stress worsens their illness. If you are a caregiver with a chronic illness it becomes even more essential that you take care of yourself first, although sadly, this doesn't always happen. Caregivers with chronic illnesses may wear themselves out because they feel they have no choice but to take on the care receiver, regardless of their own condition. Or they may be the only caregiver available. Or there may not be enough money to pay for help, or assistance by others in taking some of the burden.

I sympathize with these people. I was fortunate that Dad had the financial resources that kept me from having to give full time care, and I also protected my energy and time selfishly. Even if people have no choice but to be the primary caregiver, I urge them to get as much help as they possibly can. If there are other people who can take on the burdens of caregiving, let them do it! Work on not feeling guilty or ashamed that it is not you giving care. If there is any time that it is absolutely appropriate to be selfish, this is it. You have to look after your own needs and interests first – as much as possible.

Recently, when I began to have my medication issues, I *had* to look out for myself. I was fortunate that during this time Dad's needs weren't high. I'm not sure I could have done both – cared extensively for him and for myself. I had to be comfortable leaving his care to his caregiver, confident of how well he would be cared for.

*

What many people don't know is that even if a caregiver doesn't start out having a chronic illness, the effects of stresses (physical and emotional) from caring, if not performed mindfully and appropriately, can bring one on. People understand the detrimental effect on the body of over-use and physical stressors, so most can accept that doing too much physically can be bad. What many don't yet understand are the detrimental effects that *emotional* stressors can have on a caregiver.

The connections between body, mind, and environment have often been dismissed but are beginning to gain more attention in the scientific community. There is growing scientific evidence of something that many of us have known for a long time; that your body and your mind are interdependent and interconnected, each incapable of existing without the other, directed and affected by the body's nervous system. Most of us can cite a correlation between a stressful event or period in our lives and a tendency to get sick more often or suffer from more headaches or back pain. Think of the last time you felt overwhelmed or overburdened and your back went out, or the last family gathering that left you with a tight and painful jaw and neck, or a bad cold. We all talk about how we feel or know things in our gut – telling someone with a problem, "What does your gut tell you?" There is more going on in our body and its systems than we have been aware of.

At the biochemical level, your emotional state both affects and is affected by your hormonal state. Hormone levels in your bloodstream will affect your emotional responses, while your emotional responses also trigger hormonal releases. Stressful or traumatic situations, of course, trigger biochemical changes that are felt throughout the body. There is increasing evidence of links between attitude, external stress, and immune system functioning, and of the role played by these links in many disease processes.

Scientists are studying the connection between a perpetual stress response and the onset of inflammation and its connection to physical dysfunction. Inflammation in the body's organs, tissues, and systems, may be responsible for many of the systemic conditions plaguing our society today, such as diabetes, heart-disease and high blood pressure, and auto-immune diseases as well as neurological conditions such as Alzheimer's and Parkinson's.

Studies by the late Dr. Candace Pert, a noted neurobiologist, have shown that cancer patients who suppressed or were not consciously aware of their "negative" emotions such as resentment, anger, and grief, had demonstrably slower recovery rates than those who were more aware of their emotions and more willing to express and work through them. Another trait commonly seen in these patients was self-denial and self-sacrifice, coming from a lack of awareness of their emotional needs.

Those who were more aware of how stressors were negatively affecting them, who were more able to process the negative stress and come to terms with it, were generally healthier. Stronger immune systems and smaller tumors were the result for those patients more in touch with their needs and emotions. Apparently, chronic suppression of emotions leads to a massive upheaval in the body/mind network.

Doctors are also studying the connection between early adrenaline/fight-or-flight traumas, i.e stress, and diseases like diabetes, heart disease, and autoimmune diseases in later life. When a child's fight-or-flight adrenaline response is triggered over and over by external stress, without the chance to reset or heal itself, it can have traumatic effects on the body. Since excessive or repeated activation of the fight-or-flight response either exhausts the immune system or overstimulates it, the body is left open to infections and the possibility of autoimmune responses like Lupus and RA.

A serious illness like mine can be the somatic expression of traumatic and unsustainable stress, negative or unconscious emotions, or dysfunction. The nervous system of the body can only take so much strain and trauma before it short-circuits. When you grow up as I did, experiencing extremes in parental emotions rather than gentle, normal ups and downs in mood, you become hypervigilant. The fight-or-flight system is always activated. Our nervous systems are not accustomed to the vicissitudes of normal human behavior, and, as such, do not understand somatic middle ground. We are either on or we are off, there really isn't any "idle." Emotional and physical trauma, distress, and any other experience that exceeds what we can bear, can lay down somatic patterns in childhood that will manifest years later.

I believe the ever-present stress and tension in my family exerted an effect on my nervous system, which may have been a contributing factor to my rheumatoid arthritis. The fact that, as a child in the Christian Science religion, I was shamed for being ill, and never sure whether I would be attended to if there was a real physical emergency, also had a serious effect. Fear is a powerful emotion, and it was laid down in my system from an early age. It's hardly a surprise that my body responded to the stress of my upbringing by developing a disease that, by its very nature, is all about vigilance and enforced solidity and immovability.

The treatment technique that has helped me the most is the one developed by my therapist. It is called SPRe®; Somatic Psychological Recovery. Somatic Psychological Recovery was created to bring psychological process and its physical counterpart together for true Bodymind relief.

"Stress is a generic word to describe a very personal experience that affects everyBody differently. SPRe® helps to interpret how your body communicates, Ex. Chronic pain(head, neck, back), anxiety, digestive issues, sometimes just an overall malaise-a discomfort that doesn't have a clear explanation," says Ableson.

Her work combines physical manipulation and talk therapy and has allowed me to deal with and take care of my physical symptoms, while at the same time, exploring and integrating underlying issues both from my childhood and current experiences. You can bet that having to care for my father – the man who didn't care for me - brought out a lot of somatic symptoms. I would get migraines, suffer from TMJ, and just feel greater fatigue and pain from my RA. I was even afraid that becoming his caregiver could bring on a relapse of my disease, but by dealing with it honestly and listening to my body and creating boundaries around what I was willing to do, I was able to avoid that.

*

The nature of caregiving requires that caregivers impose too much strain and trauma on themselves every day – which too often leads to dysfunction. Being under the terrific stress that caregiving entails can bring on a lot of uncomfortable, confusing, and painful somatic responses that have a lot to do with one's emotional state. I've heard of caregivers struggling on with fibromyalgia, chronic headaches, slipped discs, chronic fatigue syndrome, rheumatoid arthritis, pneumonia...the list goes on. In fact, caregivers report suffering from chronic conditions at nearly twice the rate of non-caregivers. These conditions are all ways that the body is crying out for someone to pay attention to it and to stop the barrage of stress and exhaustion wearing it out.

At a recent party, I met a lovely but incredibly stressed woman who rattled on for fifteen minutes about her husband and his dementia, her struggles to make him comfortable, the difficult events of the past week, and the almost insurmountable problems she was facing as her husband's disease progressed. She also mentioned how stressed and short on time she was, especially lately, since she was making so many trips to the doctor in an effort to try and determine why she was feeling so sick and losing so much weight. She said this in passing, and was already moving on to another problem before I was able to process what she had just said. I cut in mid-sentence and asked her to tell me a little bit about her own health since it sounded like something serious. She said that she felt tired and sick a lot of the time and that she had lost a lot of weight in recent months, but that the doctors were having trouble figuring out what the problem was.

They had placed her on different medications in an effort to deal with the symptoms. Meanwhile, she was exhausted from caring for her husband, it was becoming apparent that another close family member would be needing care soon, and it had been only a few months since the death of another close family member, for whom she had cared briefly! It was clear this poor woman had the weight of the world on her shoulders and that her body was breaking down from the demands that were being made upon it. Her body was physically manifesting the internal and external struggles she was dealing with. For her, this was a small annoyance that was starting to become a bigger one, but she was still treating it as secondary to the problems with her husband's illness.

This woman was literally working herself to death. Even worse, she didn't seem to realize that she herself was going to need more care than her husband if she didn't somehow change what she was doing, and who, then, would care for her husband? Therein lies the problem: if we aren't aware of what could happen to us because of over-work and over-care, then we might completely break down and be useless to our care receiver. I told her about my own struggles with RA and caregiving and I urged her to spend as much time with the doctors as was needed to get help. I also gave her links to some of the local caregiving resources and suggested she get some of her extended family to help carry some of her burdens so she could get well. As caregivers, we have to be more aware, we have to accept - or get - more help, we have to fight for ourselves.

It is a well-known fact that caregivers put off doctor visits, yearly physicals, and preventative exams and tests such as mammograms and colonoscopies. They say there is not enough time, or not enough money. The number of women who have discovered they have later-stage breast cancer, for example, is heart-breakingly high. Caregivers ignore the symptoms of diabetes and heart disease far too often.

I urge caregivers to treat any mild symptoms they are feeling seriously, in order to avoid more serious ones! If they feel themselves getting sick more than normal, or just that something isn't right – get it checked out. Becoming sick with any illness, especially a chronic one, will only add to the financial, emotional, and physical difficulties of caring for a loved one. If you already *have* a chronic illness, do your best to manage it carefully. Get help.

Don't be one of the ones who end up needing more care than the care receiver!

A Few Things I Figured Out.

- Being a caregiver is the toughest job there is – illness just makes it tougher. If you already have a chronic illness and you need to meet the demands of caregiving, be as kind to yourself as possible. If you don't already have an illness, take it from me – you don't want one! Think carefully about whether you should even become a caregiver. My therapist always reminded me, when I found the going difficult, that *someone* would care for Dad if I couldn't: the county, the courts, the State, Medicaid. It may not be the best choice, but it is a choice.

- Take steps to protect yourself from over-use, over-work, and burn-out. Go to the doctor, get regular physicals, make sure you get appropriate preventative exams. Spending a little time at the doctor's now, as irritating as it might be, is better than having to go to the hospital for an extended period of time.

- Stand up for your needs and be responsible for your own self-care instead of being resentful, angry, passive aggressive, or allowing your body to break down. If you have a chronic illness, don't ignore it – you risk exacerbating your illness or developing something worse. Work your abilities and limitations into your care. Do what you can to get help in lifting your burden – you don't want to become the one who needs care! Get training from a professional on the best ways to do chores while saving your own body. Even perfectly healthy caregivers should learn how to lift with their legs to save their backs, and how to perform other tasks in a safe manner.

- If you can, find a therapist or practitioner who works with the mind/body system, there are many out there under different treatment names. Look for key words like "somatic", and "body/mind." I truly don't feel that we *can* separate the mind from the body and emotions, so we must find ways to treat both at the same time. This can be a great way to take care of yourself, relieve stress, learn how to create boundaries, and interact in the best way possible with your care receiver. Even if it's just a regular massage with a massage practitioner, you will be relieving harmful stress and adrenaline and healing your body's systems and tissues.

- There are solutions for caregivers with chronic illnesses. Ask your doctor for resources, ask your care receiver's doctor or social worker for resources. Most city, county, and state governments have assistance programs for those who aren't able to provide enough care because of physical limitations – although I would be the first to say they aren't enough. Look for a social worker who might be able to help you access local resources.

20.

Getting Out Alive.

"Life isn't about finding yourself. Life is about creating yourself." George Bernard Shaw

As individuals, most of us want to become more than who we started out being. Most of us spend our lives trying to grow and improve and achieve and accomplish more. Personally, I believe this to be one of the main points of life itself - trying to understand and improve your Self and achieving the most you can while perhaps feeling that you've made a mark on the world. There are so many, many different ways to do this, a myriad ways to make more of yourself and what you've been given: through education, basic and graduate; through spirituality or other philosophical study; self-discovery, travel, or volunteering; having or fostering a child; publishing a book; or aspiring to a better job.

Most people recognize that there are ways, even while holding down a job and coping with family, friends, and other life demands, to advance oneself in one or more of the above avenues. They pick the way that works for them, which they may end up changing, but usually by the end of the process, they have made something more of themselves. It is then common as we hit our middle years to assess what we have accomplished and whether we are fulfilled, and decide how we want to live the latter part of our lives. In my case, it would be accurate to say that my middle years hit <u>me</u> – across the head, as it were, with everything I had never achieved and would never be. After I turned 40, it seemed like nothing good was happening for me – or would ever happen.

In 1943, the psychologist Abraham Maslow published his paper, "A Theory of Human Motivation", which argues that people have a hierarchy of needs. Often depicted as a pyramid, at the bottom are basic needs – such as food, water, air, and safety, in the middle are the needs for love and belonging, next is our desire for growth and the opportunity to attain personal goals and be rewarded for our achievements. At the top is the desire for "self-actualization", self-fulfillment through pursuit of ideas and creativity for their own sake.

Although there are exceptions to Maslow's theories, I believe it is right more often than not. We want and need our basic needs to be filled, and, in fact, can't do much else but seek to fill them if they're not. However, when the first two levels are fulfilled, I think most of us have a great desire to create and attain personal goals, and receive recognition for them. We want to be more than we are. I knew I wanted to do more, to be more, to expand my life, but I wasn't sure how and felt little hope that anything would change. This feeling of depression and searching wasn't entirely new, however – it had its beginnings in my childhood.

I have always been envious of people who seem to know exactly what they want to do, or what they're good at; people who have confidence in their interests or skills, or a vocation that guides them in their life's work. As a child, I never had a clear idea of what I wanted to be, and there didn't seem to be that many people, either at school or at home, to help me determine it. I have had things I was good at and enjoyed doing, but I would never have called them a vocation. I love to read, for example, but it can be hard to find people to pay you to do it.

I have always wanted to identify my vocation and act on it – feeling as if I had the drive if only I could find a direction. I have always yearned to feel a deep calling to do a particular thing or fill a particular purpose, but have felt nothing but vague mutters about what this might be. I have wanted to achieve and be of use without having much idea of how to go about doing it.

In college, I defaulted to French as my major, with a minor in Spanish and Russian, because I had been taking French since I was in seventh grade. It was also a relatively easy major and I could get out in four years – which became even more important after I got sick. I often thought about entering the Psychology program, since I had often shown an affinity for, and skill at, counseling, but the program was long and, at my school, overcrowded.

After graduation, I worked in customer service, which I could do because it didn't require too much physical output. I proved to be quite good at it due to my empathy, attention to detail, and desire to, and pride in, helping others, but I definitely didn't feel challenged, and I wondered at dark moments if this was as far as I was going to go. In my twenties, seeking something different in my life, I trained as a massage therapist. One of the few benefits of rheumatoid arthritis, aside from convenient parking, seems to be the ability to commiserate with and assist others. I thought that my mission might be to bring massage and other healing methods to other people like me, having felt relief from my *own* illness through bodywork.

I enjoyed doing massage and, after a few years of perfecting my skills, felt I'd finally found something I was very good at that really helped people. It was really the first time I had the experience of being an expert in something, with a skill that was sought after. I enjoyed the feeling tremendously. The early desire to study counseling and psychology manifested again and I felt that part of my calling might involve helping people who were suffering from chronic diseases self-explore and get through their difficult physical and emotional situations. I wanted to be an advocate for other patients who needed better answers, better treatments, and better access to things that would help them in their struggles. I began to study techniques that integrated bodywork and counseling, while at the same time, continuing my own therapeutic process. I eventually obtained training and certification as a counselor/hypnotherapist, while continuing to practice massage.

Obviously, doing massage requires a lot of physicality, and performing it became too difficult. I suffered a recurrence of my chronic illness and couldn't do anything at all for six months, which frustrated me no end. Realizing I could no longer comfortably perform massage, and was not in a place where I had the resources to counsel others, I fell back on my remaining skill - customer service. I got a job as an assistant to a chiropractor. Once again, it was something I was good at, not something I really wanted to do. Once again, my illness had forced me to give up something I really liked doing.

When my dad got sick, I was thirty-three, and I took on the job of managing his care, a task which at least seemed to use many of my skills. Once I moved past my feelings about having to care for him, and my fear that caring for him would damage me physically, I enjoyed, and felt challenged by, taking care of Dad. I did feel like I was putting my life on hold once again to care for his. Thankfully, we eventually entered a period of his care where he was settled and comfortable and less was needed from me. After dealing with the pain medication issues when I was forty, I turned my attention yet again to what I would do with my life.

While there have been times of despair when I have wanted to give up and stop the struggle, certain things have always pulled me back. I believe that the biggest one of those things has simply been an intense desire to <u>live</u>, to go on to the next thing, the next experience, to feel and see as much as possible. I am blessed, as well, with a relatively optimistic nature, that tries to see the best in everything and everyone, and strives to experience the delights, both important and mundane, of each moment. I have also had <u>a lot</u> of therapy. Despite these things, I just kept feeling like I wanted so much *more* out of life.

Pondering what choices in further education were open to me, I realized that it was possible, even probable, that I no longer had the stamina to attempt something like grad school, another blow to future possibilities of growth. The grief from just this one realization was almost overwhelming. I really hated the inadequacy I felt – the familiar self-critique that told me that I was somehow less than the people around me because I was not changing my life or pursuing any goals or growth opportunities.

It was also during this time of self-questioning that several of the people closest to me were in the midst of some sort of renaissance or self-improvement project – either by starting new jobs or going to graduate school. They were answering a call to come up higher and be more – again, something I had always wanted for myself. It seemed as if everyone I knew was either moving up in their careers or finding their vocations, as if everyone was moving forward, expanding themselves, moving forward into the next chapter of their life; everyone but me.

Through no fault of their own, my loved ones were leaving me behind and I just could not stop feeling hopeless, pointless, boring, and stagnant. I felt so strongly that I wanted to improve myself. I was thinking about my goals, but always, frustratingly, was the reality that everything had to be within the boundaries of what I could manage physically.

Objectively, I knew that there were achievements in the past I was very proud of, times of confidence in doing the right thing or creating something special, like being Dad's caregiver, creating art, or writing. But these things were all in the past - my present felt particularly barren and uneventful. It felt as if my only claim to occupation was as a caregiver and housekeeper – not the most exalted of jobs. I felt as if I was not really providing anything worthwhile to the world, forever to be restrained and constricted both by disease and by the requirements of caregiving.

Optimistic nature aside, I have struggled for years with feelings of depression, deficiency and inferiority to others in my life because I couldn't achieve the same things professionally or physically that they could. My brain was not impaired – it is sharp, smart, and ambitious and wants to do the same stuff that everyone else is doing – but I was always battling with fatigue and physical limitations and restrictions. The mind was always willing, but the body was generally weak. How would I ever be able to better myself, accomplish things, or at the very least, feel I'd achieved something that I could be proud of and that others could respect? How could I stop feeling deficient and start finding ways to change and contribute? All in all, I felt like I was getting older, more disabled, and possibly even stupider – a glorified clerical worker with bad joints. Fortunately, help was coming in the form of a new path for my life – from a most unexpected source – a path which would ultimately lead to this book.

*

In 2009, I wrote a memoir recounting my experiences of the first five years of being Dad's caregiver as well as the story of cleaning out our family's home. I took a class on how to self-publish and market a book and decided to start a blog. I still find this a little amusing because it would be accurate to say that I'm about the last person you'd call "tech-savvy!" Everything I know about computers and the Internet is either hard won through my hunt-and-peck style of web research, totally accidental, or borrowed from someone else.

People start blogs for all sorts of reasons, but often it is because they have a story to tell, a skill to share, or even a product to advertise. Most people just like to talk about themselves – to share their stories - and blogs have served these desires admirably. In fact, there are many, *many* blogs on-line, covering all sorts of different topics and life experiences. I think it might be a little passé now to have a blog, but for a while there, it was a pretty sophisticated thing to be doing. It isn't even that hard to start one, although it is a little more challenging to actually establish and grow it. Blogs are two a penny, as most bloggers know, and making one stand out in the crowd can take a lot of work.

I had both a story to tell and a product to advertise. A book can be more attractive to publishers and just generally does better when it has an established brand or networking platform of some kind and that was to be the main purpose of the blog – a platform. At first, I posted extracts of the book, but then I began to write original material about what was happening with my father in the present moment and how I felt about it. I couldn't find an agent so I self-published the book and managed to sell a few through the blog and through Amazon. I began to attract a few more visitors to the blog, although it was still slow going.

It was important to me that the blog not just be made up of my thoughts and stories, but also be a one-stop resource for caregivers who didn't have much time to look for what they needed. I wanted the blog to be a clearinghouse for caregivers. I began to search out links to websites and other blogs and forums that I could post on the site so that people could easily find what they needed. I found organizations and events and used the blog to post interesting articles, essays, and statistics that caregivers would find helpful. I also set up a section for people to write about their own stories. I was still looking for other ways to use my time and my talents, however.

I've been told that I am a peaceful person to be around. Pondering this fact, and the fact that I had been naturally quite good at handling Dad, I decided that hospice work might be a good outlet for my talents. I began volunteering for a local hospice and bereavement program. I felt as if the opportunity to help people get through their end-of-life transitions and counsel those going through grief was a great honor, and it gave me both an identity and a purpose.

I considered it to be a job, one I prized and took very seriously, feeling as if I had found at least part of my purpose. I had designated hours that I spent in the hospice office, and I felt I was learning some important skills and making some good contacts within the field. I began to feel as if I could build a professional life on it. Unfortunately, due to budget cuts, my beloved job as a bereavement counselor/hospice worker ended when the hospice closed. It was around this time that I was going through the worst of my existential depression about what to do with my life so the timing was really bad. It didn't help that something I had so enjoyed doing, and that I was good at, was over. Knowing there was something I was good at <u>was</u> helpful, but I was at a loss as to what to do next.

Not long after this, I noticed that my blog appeared to be gaining popularity, either through longevity (I'm sure), or improved material that people enjoyed reading (I hope.) I began to see that other, bigger, blogs and sites were linking to, or mentioning, mine. I found another big caregiving site that had written an article about some of the best dementia blogs - including mine, which was exciting.

After I had an essay published in an anthology sold by a large caregiver support website, they asked me to be a guest on one of their weekly webcasts to talk about the subject of my essay. This was followed a month later by another invitation to tell my caregiver story on another webcast. I felt as if I was entering the wider world of writers, bloggers, and caregiver advocates – and that my work actually meant something.

The crowning achievement was being notified by Healthline.com (a huge health website that I had never heard of) that I was one of their 25 Best Dementia Blogs of 2012. To say I was amazed was a massive understatement. I never dreamed that a major website would not only *see* my blog, but think it belonged with twenty-four other, undoubtedly successful and professional, blogs.

I have won things in my day, gotten good grades or succeeded in a job, even been celebrated for achievements or just for being me. But I can safely say that this award meant more to me than almost anything that came before. To be validated for my work - for my writing as well as the care I put into the information and the support I supply in my blog – that was huge, especially since it came in this particularly dark time of my life. I felt as if I had created something out of my pain and sorrow and desire to matter that was making some sort of impact. Learning how to promote my blog and network with all the social media outlets now available gave me a certain sort of confidence. The connections I made through the blog were leading not only to those commendations, which I was happy to receive, but also to my future.

In the early part of 2012, through my Internet searches, I found an organization similar to the Alzheimer's Foundation that needed help. The Lewy Body Dementia Association, a non-profit organization that provided information and services about Lewy body dementia to sufferers and their caregivers, had a hot line for caregivers who needed information, support, or just a compassionate ear. I began to volunteer for them as a counselor, a job that I could do from home and on my own time, that was manageable with my disease. I also began volunteering for another hospice organization doing bereavement groups and counseling.

One of my goals has always been to keep studying and reading as much as I could about dementia and caregiving so that I would have the correct information and comfort for the people who came to me. I found myself drawing on this knowledge as well as my personal experiences with Dad. I felt that I was finally unearthing the achievements I felt were within me – the work I desperately wanted to do. As I met and talked to more and more caregivers, I began to realize that, completely unsuspectingly, I had found my vocation. I realized that I was using what I had learned as a caregiver, my natural compassion and empathy, and all of the study and research to create a career for myself – what I called caregiver advocacy. I was creating a profession out of the most surprising material – Dad's illness, and my response to it.

*

Out of suffering and darkness came my life's work. Dad's dementia, along with everywhere I had been employed and everything else I had gone through, or learned, combined to make me very good at what I was doing. It brought together all of my skills and past jobs: counseling and customer service, empathy, clerical and financial training, writing and research, and, especially, caregiving. It was the perfect amalgamation of everything I've experienced, learned, and studied. Most importantly for my self-esteem, I began to once again feel of value and use. I went from feeling stagnant and deficient in skills and self-worth to a feeling of sufficiency, positive self-worth, and discovery. Caregiving - the very thing that I thought was such a challenge and struggle in my life - would be the thing that would bring me the most contentment and self-satisfaction.

How do we endure, and how do we take our suffering and turn it into something that will give to us instead of taking something away? However we can. Sometimes we are granted the strength and the grace to transform something negative – in my case, chronic illness and Dad's dementia – into something positive. Eventually, over time, I made my way through the dark place into a much happier one. I have found myself and my vocation, and I try to be more aware of tying my self-esteem and feelings of sufficiency to what I have achieved as compared to others. (It does help that I now can claim to be a published writer – something I really never could have imagined being! And yes, I do find it funny that it was the blog and not the book that ended up taking off, although the growing popularity of the blog has led to a few more book sales.)

I am still experiencing the ups and downs of life. I continue to explore ways to come to terms with the restrictions and requirements of my illness and how I can go on living around it. I still struggle with what aging with a chronic illness means to me, and trying to process the resentment and bitterness that I feel about it. This is something I feel I will be working on for the rest of my life. Going through my dark night of the Soul was not a comfortable time, but I am proud of myself that I kept going, and made the effort to create something for myself. I believe in Maslow's pyramid, and in the thought that we need to become something more – strive for personal goals. In the midst of suffering, I found a purpose – a vocation -and a way to make a hard thing mean something.

It does make me shake my head bemusedly when I think of the circumstances of finding such a vital part of myself. It always gives me pause when people thank me for my help with their suffering/dementia problems/caregiving woes/grief/et al. and I say, "That's okay, I love doing it." Inevitably, I then qualify my statement with, "Well, I don't love it, I don't love that something terrible is happening to you and you need help, but I do like being of use." People seem to understand, fortunately. The point is, I truly don't think I would be the person I am today if my father had not become ill and required my help. Dementia has been the gateway to my sense of purpose.

It has led to confidence in my counseling skills, a career as a writer and blogger, and a place in the wider community of caregiver advocates, bereavement counselors, patient counselors, and dementia specialists. I was asked to come up higher, to have the courage to work through issues like anger and resentment, and to allow my Self to expand. As a result, my whole world has expanded, while I have watched my father's gently contract.

And I always feel like, if *I* can do it, anyone can do it. Anyone out there who feels as deficient as I sometimes do, who feels that they've been handed a bad deal because of a chronic illness, or a loved one's dementia, or who feels worn out and bitter by the demands of caregiving – those people can create something for themselves, as well. There are a lot of great blogs, forums, Facebook pages, and books written by and for caregivers. People just like me who found their situation intolerable and found relief in writing about it or telling others or helping caregivers. I urge everyone to see if you can create something special for yourself out of your hardship.

*

We all deserve to feel that we are worthwhile, that our lives matter as much as the next person's. Caregivers especially must allow themselves to believe that their lives also have value and that they deserve to have those lives, with all the attendant growth, transformation, relationships, and experiences. If they don't, they risk starting to feel that they are deficient somehow. I define deficiency in terms of self-esteem, self-worth, and personal growth and it is something I am intimately acquainted with.

I believe that if one is not feeling sufficiently valued, challenged, fulfilled, or engaged – if one is not reaching for the top of Maslow's pyramid - then one may start feeling deficient. This underlying belief system may begin to negatively affect and define a caregiver. A caregiver, by definition, spends much of their time and energy taking care of another's life besides their own. When it comes to successfully living their own lives, they face unavoidable restrictions and restraints in terms of lack of time, energy, and emotional resources and stability.

It can be very hard to find the time do any of the other activities that people normally do to improve their minds, careers, lives, and well-being. If it appears that friends or colleagues are growing and changing and reaping the benefits of time and energy to go to school, or change jobs, or improve themselves in some other fashion while one is still stuck giving care, it can lead to depression and despair. During your time as a caregiver, your peers, friends, or family members may grow, have a family, go to grad school, get a new job, travel, and otherwise enlarge themselves, while you're still caring: researching new meds, wiping bottoms, hand-feeding, and learning creative ways to gently distract your charge from holding a garage sale of your shoes, or calling a taxi to take them to visit their mother – who's been dead for twenty years.

As a caregiver, committed to the care and feeding of another for an unspecified length of time, it can be hard not to watch the activities and achievements of the people around you and not feel like yours are distinctly lacking. I speak personally when I say that it can be emotionally devastating if this one thing, caregiving, is all your life seems to be, for the present and the foreseeable future. I have had to struggle repeatedly with feelings of low self-esteem and hopelessness during the times I had no energy for anything but my duties. What I wanted was to be out in the world advancing my education, gaining respect and knowledge, making a difference.

What I had was a father with dementia, rheumatoid arthritis, and no time or energy for anything else.

Between 40-70% of family caregivers experience depression. A study found that one in four caregivers have contemplated suicide more than once a year. If it feels as if people are moving on around you, while you remain where you are, you may have to deal with any feelings of anger, depression, low self-esteem, and deficiency that can burgeon up. The perceptions of caregivers towards themselves can become damaging to good mental and emotional health and well-being. This, when added to the fact that caregivers are expected by society to submerge their lives, needs, and goals to those of their loved one, can cause a heavy emotional burden for caregivers.

Giving care, no matter the reason or illness, can be a long game – you'll most likely be caring for many years. The lack of specificity about when your tour of duty as a caregiver will be ending can make it very difficult to manage what you want to achieve in your own life, especially if you are a younger caregiver like I am. After all, there's no clock by which dementia or most other illnesses runs, and it is impossible to know when that clock will stop. Caregivers who are in their thirties, forties, and fifties may look ahead at their own lives, measured by the deterioration of another's, and wonder if by the time they're finally free to live and achieve and accomplish, it will be too late for them.

Older caregivers have probably already had the chance to develop their lives, interests, and careers. However, in this day and age, people switch careers and occupations several times over their lives, or they may come late in life to the occupation or vocation that truly suits them. Giving that up to give care will be difficult. These older caregivers may also wonder when they will be able to pick up the threads of their own lives, or whether they will be physically and mentally able to do so when their duties end. All caregivers, no matter what age, want to do what is right, but we are sacrificing our lives.

Granted, caregiving can be a noble profession and a worthwhile thing to be doing with our time and energy. None of us are one-dimensional, however, and for most people, caregiving is not enough to stretch or fulfill their mental and physical capacities. What we do and achieve with those capacities can matter so much to our emotional well-being and satisfaction with our lives. I believe that there are ways to use all of our capabilities, improve our minds, make a difference, or expand our horizons – the key is how we do it and the scale in which we do it.

Caregivers want the same things as any other individual on this planet; to live the lives they want, to improve and expand their experiences and accomplishments, and to feel like they've made an impact, some sort of impression on the world. The problem is finding the time, energy, and capacity necessary to do these things when so much of it is already spoken for. Caregivers must learn to start keeping s*omething* back for themselves – time to themselves, friends, a hobby, a few hours of work or volunteering, or a course of study.

*

If you are giving care, chances are you don't have that much time to expand your career or take that promotion. In fact, giving care may be the only employment you have the time to do. If this is the case, keep in mind that caregiving is, in fact, a professional job – why not treat it as such? Caregivers who regard themselves as trained professionals are much less vulnerable to self-esteem problems than those who regard themselves as relatives.

Caregiving requires patience and determination, the will to face challenges, the ability to problem solve and make decisions, and a lot of other skills – a combination that any employer would feel lucky to have in an employee. Caregivers are health care professionals, financial managers, clerical experts, tax pros, behavioral specialists, and nutritionists. We are doing the jobs of professional nurses, accountants, counselors, and financial planners, all rolled into one. We are executives!

Sadly, our government isn't quite at the enlightened level of other countries that offer family caregivers pay and benefits for their time and energy, but I believe we are moving that way. Until that time, believe that the services you are offering are worth the full pay and benefits that "professional" caregivers get. (Keeping in mind, of course, that they don't get paid very well, either!) I strive to feel like a professional at what I do, not only as a caregiver advocate but as a caregiver. The research and studying I have done has made me more knowledgeable about my dad's disease and how to care for him, and learning how to run his affairs gave me skills and knowledge I might not otherwise have had.

I encourage caregivers to consider themselves professionals and train themselves accordingly. Many health clinics, hospitals, senior centers, area agencies on aging, and local chapters of national organizations now offer classes on how to give good health care; manage financial, business, and legal affairs; physically assist and entertain the aging and ill; and how to help others who are embarking on the care journey. There are many who could benefit from your knowledge and experience in these areas: consider offering them to organizations who help others.

You may not have time to go to full time graduate school, but there are now a lot of on-line education programs and low-residence trainings and certification programs. You could potentially earn certificates in psychology, social work, healthcare, or eldercare. I have done a great deal of research and study on-line, finding organizations that offer study and training courses to do in my own time, like a thanatology (death and dying) training course through The Thanatology Association. I also read a great deal and have expanded my knowledge and abilities just by reading a range of books on healthcare, aging, illness and dementia, and end of life topics.

You might want to study something completely out of the realm of healthcare and caregiving, in which case there are a huge number of low-attendance, on-line, and continuing education courses available on any number of subjects. Most cities have at least one community college that offers continuing education; many cities have colleges and universities that run similar programs. Creative writing, literature, poetry, drawing, art, photography, music, finance, computers, and more are all available through this kind of program. Learn more about social media or computer programming, become a writer, or take accounting classes. Usually, these courses require only a few hours a week including study time.

You may not be able to take on a high-power career but there are a lot of volunteer opportunities. There are many organizations that are crying out for help in many different areas, with the added benefit that much of the work can be done in your home. Start a support group – real or virtual. When I found the LBDA and learned that, with a little bit of training, I could work from home by counseling other caregivers, I was thrilled.

Volunteering as a bereavement counselor with a local hospice and grief program also gave me the opportunity to make calls from home. I found that volunteering for that hospice program as a hospice volunteer took only a few hours of my time a week for patient visits, with some travel time, and it got me out of the house! At last, I had a job and an occupation that made me feel good about myself.

You probably don't have a great deal of time for hobbies but there are so many that can be done at home with the right supplies and a little room. There are thousands of on-line groups through which to connect with people that share interests and abilities, as well as how-to videos and descriptions. Don't underestimate the benefit of creating art and making craft projects with your care receiver, who might still really enjoy the chance to scrapbook, paint, work with clay, knit, quilt, etc. Put aside some time for yourself alone to spend time on art projects that interest and fulfill you.

Granted, travel can be difficult when one is giving care, but by arranging respite care, small trips may be taken. If no respite is available, once again the Internet is available. Going on-line to explore different countries and cultures is easy – there is a wealth of information, pictures, and even on-line museum sites. Invest in a language learning program – it is quite easy to find literature in other languages now for reading practice. There are many good travelogues and travel memoirs now, as well as on-line magazines and websites. Now is the time to plan, and perhaps save for, the big trip you may take when your care receiver no longer needs your help.

Many people find a creative, and emotional, outlet in writing about their caregiving journey. There are countless blogs detailing regular people's experiences; it is not necessary to be a professional writer to share your story. Start a blog, write a book, or submit articles and essays to other blogs, websites, and forums. Many websites now welcome guest bloggers. Start a journal that you could someday turn into a book – many caregivers have done this. Even if you don't write a book, you will have had a processing outlet, and a record of everything that happened to you. While there are already many memoirs about caregiving, written from the perspective of caregivers, your experience is unique and it may help someone else to read about it.

Some sort of social life is also important. One of the first things that happens to caregivers is isolation: friends drift away or don't know how to help, available social time is curtailed, fatigue and/or resentment interfere with a caregiver reaching out, and people have busy lives. If possible, we must try to avoid this so that when the caregiving duties end, we still have somewhat of a social connection. My own sibling found it impossible to give me much support and companionship and I think one of the reasons I became so quickly involved with my then-boyfriend, Charlie, was because I felt isolated and frightened by my new caregiving duties. If I hadn't had Charlie, and my therapist, to talk to and spend time with, I probably would have become very isolated.

As a caregiver, you must maintain some sort of social network that will sustain you during caregiving and after it. It is possible that old friends *do* want to help and remain in your life, but don't know how; if you are bad at asking for help or letting them know what you need, acknowledge that and reach out. Admittedly, old friends from before may drop away, but new friends are waiting to be discovered: in support groups, forums, book groups, and by pursuing new interests. It is also possible to rediscover old friendships after caregiving ends if you reach out. Allowing yourself to become completely isolated and friendless serves nobody, and may harm your health and ability to give good care.

I still cherish some of my old friendships – people who continue to stick with me during this long journey with Dad. I have made new friends and contacts through my support groups and my writing and my work, and, of course, after breaking up with Charlie, I met someone new and got married. I maintained a relationship with my therapist, as well, who knows my life intimately and who nurtures me in a parental caring way. I have the supports I need to continue doing what I must for Dad, and I also have friends who can help me forget my duties.

*

Imagine my surprise when I looked around and realized life had happened around me, and in my struggles I had achieved more growth and transformation than I realized. Once I looked, it became easy to see how much my life had bloomed. Surprisingly, all the little things I was doing

As I learned when I broke off the five year relationship that started when I moved in with Dad, and then began dating again – you *can* live your own life while being a caregiver. In fact, you must. By creating a new purpose for myself, increasing my writing skills, and getting out to meet new people, I have managed to maintain my own life next to my life as a caregiver. Even if it means making compromises, cutting a few corners, or having to create something entirely new that works for you – you have to date, or have a relationship, or create, or work, or have a child, or build a house, or get married, or have a significant friendship, or write a book, or express that you are alive in some way.

You must have something that is yours. You must use those talents and skills that have nothing to do with caregiving. In addition, those talents and skills that are all about caregiving must be appreciated and seen for the professional skills they are. While it may be difficult to find the time, energy, space, money, self-capacity, etc., I firmly believe it is possible, and not only possible but of primary importance.

One of the reasons it is important to keep something for yourself *during* your caregiving journey is because your life will hopefully be continuing on for years to come *after* it. Whether you are at the beginning, in the middle, or at the end of your long road, no matter how old you are, it is important to keep in mind that it will someday reach an end. What will happen then? Someday, there will be a life after caregiving; living, maintaining, and developing one's own life in the duration is your right.

Most caregivers perform their duties anywhere from one year to more than fifteen, and since giving care can be so time consuming and all-encompassing, many caregivers find themselves giving up a lot – friends, hobbies, activities, travel, careers, job advancement, and even financial security – in order to perform their duties. The entire family and care structure may be focused on the care-taker and their needs, without much thought, discussion, or planning for when that will no longer be the case.

What do you want your life to look like when you regain it? I don't feel that being a caregiver has kept me from getting on with my life, nor that the end of it will cause me to be at a loss, since I have my work and many other activities and family to help give my life meaning. I do feel that there are definitely certain activities and bigger choices that I can't make until my father is gone. However, I have spent some time thinking about what those activities and choices might be, something I encourage other caregivers to do as they reach an end.

I think it is important for all caregivers to think about the future regardless of whether one is just at the beginning of the caregiving journey, halfway through, or approaching the end. The duties of caregiving and the needs of another arise and cancel out everything else for a year or two years or ten years. But after the duties are done, and the affairs have been settled, and the family has gone home - there may now be a chance to do something different, a chance to move on with one's life; perhaps not exactly in the ways one had planned, but in new ways.

Many caregivers report succumbing to a serious illness or illnesses after the loss of their care receiver. Perhaps this is because they finally have the time, internal space, and capacity to listen to the physical problems that they have been suppressing from stress and lack of time. One woman I spoke to whose husband had died a few years previously said that she spent some time in the hospital after his death; suffering from everything the flu to ear and brain infections.

There have even been caregivers who have followed their loved ones into death, although this usually happens with older caregivers. Keeping in mind the very real chance of serious physical dysfunction at the end of caregiving if the body has been pushed too far may help you pay attention to what the body is telling you while you are still caring. If it has proven impossible to care for personal health issues while giving care, and serious physical problems have resulted, try to recognize that now is the time to focus on your own care and health and pay attention to what your body may be telling you.

To me, caregiving, and living with RA, has been all about learning to live with the things I can't control, while putting my energy into affecting the things I can. I've spoken elsewhere of the importance of listening to your body's limits, especially when it is strained to breaking point. When you slow down, the body will see its chance and take it, and the repercussions of this can be serious.

We must take responsibility for ourselves and make sure we get out alive.

I'm closing in on the finish of my role as a caregiver, although I have no real idea when those responsibilities will end. The way my father's disease is going, it could be one year or three years or seven years before he is gone and I no longer have to consider him and his needs in most of the decisions that I make. I am on-call twenty-four hours a day and seven days a week and I am never far from my phone – even when I'm on vacation.

While my husband and I have discussed moving to different states for job opportunities for him and a better climate for me - until Dad is gone I don't feel free to live anywhere else but here. I wouldn't feel comfortable not being close by in order to monitor his care and well-being and deal with his business affairs. I also have to limit my volunteer and work commitments in order to have adequate time to deal with his affairs and his needs, and I am well aware that when we approach the end, I will most likely be dedicating most of my time and energy to his end of life process.

How can we ensure that we are able to move past our mission as a caregiver when the time comes, into a happy, functional life of our own? I believe one way is by having some sort of plan for what is going to come after. Recently, I have started to see people talking more about what will happen at the end of caregiving; either in books or on forums and blogs. They are going past the end of life options, the practical issues, and the grief and talking about what caregivers are supposed to do with themselves once it happens.

I realize how difficult it can be to allot mental and emotional space to what may seem like frivolous dreaming when so much is currently required of you, but it could be a lifesaver. Imagining what you might like to do, where you might like to go, even ways you may wish to change your residence or job can give you hope and something to focus on during your duties. Having something to dream about or look forward to can provide a necessary emotional stability. Sometimes, just the act of planning gives you a foundation for hope and a structure of information and possibilities to tap into when the time comes. Even if none of these plans materialize, odds are they might lead to something else that will prove to be what works for you.

It is entirely possible that few of the plans you're making will come about, but it is the planning that really matters, if only for your psyche. When I was cleaning out Dad's house, I gave myself a deadline and arranged a trip to Hawaii for just after that goal month. Having something to look forward to, as well as an incentive to get the job done, really helped me to navigate through an intense, difficult process.

*

The other kinds of plans that really matter are practical ones. Do you have plans for the time after caregiving? Do you have any savings or a retirement plan? Are you financially secure or will you have to go back to work? Will you even be able to get another job in your field after taking years off? Social security benefits are based on lifetime earnings and if there are years without earnings, it brings down your wage average, which reduces benefits.

The Social Security system does not yet recognize informal caregiving as real work, unfortunately, so no benefits will accrue. Caregivers who take time off work face a reduction in benefits upon retirement. Other countries are beginning to recognize the importance of providing retirement benefits for family caregivers, but our country has a ways to go before such a positive arrangement is made here. Therefore, it falls to us to make preparations for our own futures. Do you have your own health insurance, or long-term care insurance? If you have been living with your care receiver, do you have an unencumbered home to remain in? It is so important to have some sort of plan.

We must also consider, and plan for, the *emotional* impact on us of the death of our care receiver. Not only will you be feeling the grief and loss of that person, you will also be feeling the grief and loss of your role in that person's life and your place in the world. Until now, most days have been relatively familiar and slipping into your place and duties as the caregiver has become second nature. When that place is no longer necessary, it may leave a hole.

Many caregivers feel lost after the death of their care-taker, stating that they don't know who they are anymore when it's not in relationship to their loved one; they may feel as if they no longer have a purpose in life. When one has gotten up each day and performed the same jobs over and over and focused one's life solely on the task of caring, it can be difficult to know what to do next. One's purpose was clear and life had meaning.

The familiar, even if it is difficult, is comforting – loss of the familiar and loss of purpose can lead to physical dysfunction and emotional difficulties and depression. A good way to deal with the grief of losing one's care receiver *and* one's role as caregiver is to have a trusted professional or other individual to talk to. Some caregivers find this outlet in support groups where they are able to speak to individuals who have already gone through the loss of their care-taker. Having this kind of discussion can be invaluable in showing what that life can look like, that other meanings and roles can be discovered, and that caregiving ends – because it does.

I am sure that when Dad dies, I will still suffer the bewilderment, guilt, loss of purpose, and other problems inherent in the loss of a parent and the loss of my role. However, I will have established a foundation of awareness, self-care, personal interests and pastimes, and people that will help support me and carry me through the end. Start practicing now – both what you want to do and who you want to be. Look for that relationship that will give you strength and support. The dreaming and the planning start now, even if only in the smallest way, with no guilt allowed. You can have a life, but you have to put aside the resources and the time to create it.

Believe me when I say that I know how difficult it can be to find the time to do something for yourself when you are giving care. I was fortunate enough to have financial resources that allowed me to hire others to help me with Dad – resources that most caregivers do not have. I know what most caregivers deal with in terms of lack of time, energy, and resources. However, I also know that keeping some sort of self-validating, self-esteem boosting, mind-expanding, capacity-stretching, skill-using time and space is absolutely essential to prevent burn-out, compassion fatigue, and depression.

A Few Things I Figured Out.

- Changing healthcare and technology are extending lives; people with dementia can live for twenty years or more. The prevalence of diseases like MS, ALS, Parkinson's, and diabetes creates more people needing care for longer periods of time. All of these things can lead to an extended, difficult, self-worth challenging tour of duty for a caregiver. In order to avoid burning out during this time, you must hold on to something for yourself. Your life matters just as much as your care receiver's and you have the right to live and develop it.

- Don't fall into the trap of focusing on the things you're not achieving, the heights you're not scaling, the feeling that life is passing you by, or that you feel less than others. Take charge of your own self-worth and whatever feelings of deficiency you may have, and be proud of what you can do. It took me a long time to realize that I was using every skill I'd ever learned, both before caregiving and after, to create a profession that I was really proud of – caregiver advocacy.

- There are more and better health and caregiving classes being offered by local governments, hospitals, facilities, senior organizations, and non-profits than ever before. Take advantage of these opportunities to receive more advanced training. Think of yourself as a valued professional, performing a necessary and challenging job – because you are! You are a professional caregiver – an asset and a highly knowledgeable and qualified individual.

- While it's true that there may not be time and money enough to do something like complete an advanced degree, or become a CEO, there are ways we can improve ourselves. Reading and studying independently, online classes, continuing education, and low-residency trainings or certifications are all good ways to educate oneself. Starting a small, or on-line, business in one's home or volunteering are good ways to use one's skills and possibly make money.

- Starting a blog or Facebook page, writing a memoir, or being a guest blogger are great ways to expand oneself. Signing up for book groups as a way of being social and expanding your library can help. Learning a language and visiting on-line museums and travel sites can temporarily take the place of travel. I don't have the stamina at the moment to get an advanced degree in healthcare or counseling, but I read, take training courses, and I volunteer. Allow your creativity and positive self-worth to flow. Get busy.

21.

Good Grief.

"So it's true, when all is said and done, grief is the price we pay for love." E.A. Bucchianeri

There are so many different types of grief and loss and bereavement. There are some that everyone will experience, like the loss of a parent; some that only certain people will go through depending on life events, like the loss of a spouse, or personal loss through disease; and some that only people living with dementia can experience, like the grief of anticipation. I have no experience yet with the loss of a spouse, although I can imagine, and have witnessed, how difficult an event it is.

The death of my mother hit my father hard. Although he returned to work and his life in his Church, he was never the same person. His brief relationship with Janet brought him back into the world for a time, but after she left, he essentially shut down - retreating into his grief, his house, his few interests, and his own company. I sometimes think his dementia was a natural result of his depression and disconnection with the external world. Grief is a response to love, and the loss of the object of that love. Grief is a natural, instinctual, healthy emotional process that humans have been experiencing for thousands of years. Lately, however, it has lost some of its naturalness. Grieving has become something of an uncomfortable topic in our society.

We don't quite know how to talk about it, or what to do about it, and we don't always acknowledge how important it is to mental health to be able to grieve. There is no denying that Elisabeth Kubler-Ross and her five stages of death and dying – denial, anger, bargaining, depression, and acceptance – put a more comprehensible face on grief. Her work brought the concepts of grief as an acceptable process into the forefront of the mainstream, and helped give the average person a vocabulary for the difficulties and emotions with which they were dealing. Even with her work, however, we are still, as a society, deeply uncomfortable with grief – what it is, what it does, what it means, and the needs of those experiencing it.

It is important to be aware that Kubler-Ross worked with dying patients, not people who were grieving, and she noted that there was no specific sequence for the stages and that they were not the *only* emotions that could be felt. Unfortunately, they have still entered the lexicon of the general public as being the definitive way to experience grief because of a loss, narrowing people's understanding and expectations of the process. Experts who have continued studying grief and loss since Kubler-Ross have begun to suggest new models and concepts about what grieving is – even exploring the fact that some people don't seem to experience much grief at all and are coping perfectly well. The basic truth about grieving is that it is a unique process and one that is as individual as the individual who experiences it.

The main goal that bereavement counselors strive for is to normalize grief for those experiencing it. This essentially means telling people that since grief can look and feel like a lot of different things, and have both emotional and physical components, there is no right or wrong way to grieve. I tell people that it can manifest in many different ways, physically and mentally, and that there is no ordered progression of feelings – they can occur front to back, back to front, repeatedly, or not at all.

Grief can make you feel crazy, it can make you think and do strange things, cry or not cry. An individual can feel loss physically - as pain, discomfort, stiffness, lack of or excessive appetite, forgetfulness, and confusion. This is not the time to be making big decisions, signing contracts, moving house, or even travelling, if possible, because of the risk of physical, emotional, or even financial, harm.

Since no two relationships are the same, no experience of grief will be the same. We can never know exactly what another person is feeling or going through, even if they've been in a similar situation, experienced a death or some other grief. When counseling, I always say that I've felt something of what they're feeling, or, that I've been in a similar situation but that there is no way I could know exactly what they're feeling. Each person's situation is unique – there is no "normal."

*

Dad is firmly ensconced in the Adult Family Home that is now his home. A few years ago, we began to notice that going out into the world was causing him too much agitation, so we made the decision that the time for casual trips had stopped. At some point, almost every dementia sufferer becomes too uncomfortable and over stimulated by the world outside and can no longer leave their home. Dad was no different.

Dad went from escaping his facility to wander for miles and looking forward to long drives in the car to being essentially housebound. He no longer craves escape, nor does this once highly fit and physical man seem over-eager to even walk down the hall. He can no longer walk as he did in his prime, with long, strong, confident strides - muscles, joints, tendons all working as they should, receiving the appropriate messages from his brain. Now, when he does walk, he shuffles carefully, uncertainly, confused as to exactly where the ground is in relation to his feet.

He leans back unexpectedly - his body anxious to find a chair or somewhere to rest – so unexpectedly that his caregivers must walk behind him to make sure he doesn't fall. It is entirely possible that his brain no longer transmits or receives the correct messages about height, and distance, and pounds per square inch, and where the feet are going, and that the next foot needs to be lifted up in preparation for a step. The Parkinson's part of his Lewy body dementia has ensured that his muscles, joints, and ligaments are no longer experiencing proprioception, flexibility, or the ability to bear weight.

He spends his days quietly, sleeping, eating when told to, then dozing on the recliner in his room. Day after day, his routine is virtually unchanging, uneventful, and always takes place at home. I make a point of saying all of this so that it is clear that there is no chance that at any random moment, he is going to be anywhere else but in his home, quietly passing the day. Which is what why it is so strange that I keep seeing him, everywhere I go.

I will be driving down a road and see from behind a lanky figure, perhaps with white hair, walking along the sidewalk, and think, "That's Dad!" Actually, it is less a conscious thought than an impulse. We all have bodily recognition of someone we know – a way of recognizing people even if we can't see them very well. A sign that the person you are near is familiar to you in a deeply important way. In these moments of a sighting, I can feel my heart briefly, almost physically, yearn towards the person I am seeing, until a few seconds elapse and my conscious brain takes over and assures me that there is no way that my father would be striding briskly down a street in Seattle.

I will go into the drug store to pick something up, and see someone next to me in the aisle, a man perhaps, and something about that person - a way of standing, the position of a shoulder, their hair or clothes -will bring up that same deep feeling of recognition, that quick thought of, "That's Dad!" And, of course, it won't be, can't be, my dad, standing in the candy aisle of the drug store, pondering on what type of treat to buy. (Although, to be honest, my father was often to be found in the candy aisle, deciding what treat to get, which would end up in his desk or dresser drawer for months before he ate it.)

It even happens sometimes with women, if something about their posture, or physical presence, or coloring reminds me at all of Dad. There is that quick, flushed feeling of recognition, a certainty that I am in proximity to a person who has deep meaning to me. And then there's an equally quick realization that it's not who I thought. And all of this happens inside of a few seconds.

It keeps happening, over and over. Which makes me wonder - are we just hard wired to seek the image of someone we know in someone with similar physical traits? Is it a function of loss or the long grief of my father's condition? Is this a phenomenon common to other caregivers? Does it happen only to people who have lost or are losing a loved one? I don't know. I haven't heard anyone else talking about it, but then maybe it's something people keep to themselves in fear of seeming a little nuts.

It's been over twenty years since my mom died and I guess I still a flash of her when I see a petite woman with short, dark brown hair and laughing brown eyes. It can be as small a flash as seeing the shape of her hand in someone else's. So maybe I shouldn't feel surprised that my brain seeks out someone loved once but no longer around. It makes me think of alternate realities, other possibilities that might have been, where his life wouldn't have shrunk down to his chair and his room and his caregiver having to feed him his lunch, and it's the *actual* reality that seems strange, not the imagined one. It's all an illusion and the world where my father has been ravaged by dementia doesn't exist. These thoughts definitely make me sad.

I think I have been grieving the loss of my father since the day I walked into his cold, cluttered house and saw how he had been living. It's been ten long years, now that I've watched him gradually disappear. I stretch my memory back to those years when I lived with him and he was still somewhat lucid and could move and run and Rollerblade – and I can hardly believe they happened.

I suspect it is just something that comes along with loss – and not just loss by death – it can also be loss of the person you knew. Seeing the ghost of my dad isn't particularly disturbing or devastating, just a little weird. It happens maybe once a month. I feel it, remember where he actually is, and then I drive on, or keep walking through the store, or generally move on with my day. It does make me think, however, about Dad and how his day is going, and how if things had been very, very different, it is entirely possible that he *would* have been walking down the street, or picking up something at the store, or running an errand, or eating in a restaurant.

Bereavement as a caregiver can be uniquely difficult because there are so many complicating factors. Many people who are personally experiencing dementia in a loved one refer to it as "the long, slow good-bye." The phrase refers to the fact that a loved one is being taken little by little, and will most likely be completely gone, long before their actual death. There is a term for the feelings this type of event engenders – anticipatory grief – whereby a person anticipates the loss and can begin grieving it before it is a reality, i.e. my dad sightings. While this creates the space for someone to grieve over time, without being overwhelmed by bereavement as at a final death, it can also be exhausting to have the situation strung out for so long.

There is another term that applies to this situation – "ambiguous loss." Pauline Boss writes about it clearly: "Perceiving loved ones as present when they are physically gone, or perceiving them as gone when they are physically present, can make people feel helpless and thus more prone to depression, anxiety, and relationship conflicts. Those who suffer the loss have to deal with something very different from ordinary, clear-cut loss." Dementia removes loved ones from us mentally and emotionally, but leaves their physical shell to still care for. It can be difficult to grieve and say good-by to someone when they are still there to physically remind you of what once was. It is a process that can be exhausting and it lasts as long as the life of your loved one.

Having the sightings I described above makes me feel like I'm practicing - practicing for the time when my father is no longer in the world. I feel like I am practicing grieving, because each time it happens, I feel a little pinch of sadness – and the ambiguity of my situation. I think it will be a little easier than my mother's death, having had all this practice, so to speak, but I imagine I will still feel grief at his final passing. I guess I just don't want to lose my father – so I pretend I see him everywhere I go.

At some point, the ambiguous loss will become unambiguous – absolutely definite – and I will be able to move on. I know this. Until that time, however, I have no closure around the situation. Closure would definitely be easier for those of us who care for a loved one with dementia. It would also be easier for those around us, who may not realize that we are mourning every day.

*

As I have reason to know, the loss of a parent is a unique type of grief. For those of us caring for a parent, contemplating the death of that parent can be difficult; not only because of our love for that person, but also due to the loss of one's history as known uniquely by one's parent. The death of parents is almost a loss of self

– it's a loss of part of your story because nobody remembers your history, your childhood, like a parent. After the loss of a parent, it can be hard to remember that you were once part of an organism – a system – created of people who knew you and loved you and were part of you.

A year ago, I brought my mother-in-law, Nan, to my father's Adult Family Home over the Thanksgiving holiday and introduced her to my father. Miraculously, Dad was alert and in a good mood, following along with our conversation with his caregivers, laughing when we laughed. As we spoke about the visit later at dinner, Nan told me how much I looked like Dad, that we had the same eyes and that I shared his coloring, comments that I was pleased to hear.

It wasn't until a little bit later that I felt the full effect of the visit and could explore the phrases Nan had used and what they might mean to me. I never hear comments like this anymore. They are words people use casually all the time, off-handedly noting a resemblance between child and parent. They were words I had grown hungry to hear without realizing. What is just a social pleasantry to most people becomes poignant and important to those who no longer experience it: it creates and affirms a relationship between you and your parents, anchors you in time and space within a family structure. It caught me off guard, how much it meant to me to hear that I resembled my father. She witnessed the two of us together and commented on our shared traits, the things that related us to each other. I wasn't prepared for the depth of emotion I felt.

I've lived so long with the unconventionality of my life that I sometimes forget about its oddities, about what it is lacking, and about the sadness in it. Sometimes it seems like the man I take care of and visit and make decisions for is just an idea called my father. I talk about him as my father, and that's how everyone refers to him, but it's still very abstract. Only Paul, my husband, and one or two of my good friends have even met him. It's not as if I'm ashamed of him or his dementia, but the occasion to introduce him to someone important just doesn't arise very often. He's more of a distant relation, in a strange way, and I'm so accustomed to how things are, that it feels like I have no parents left at all.

Sadly, there is no substitute for the family you were born with, who know you, good and bad, happy and sad. I feel strongly that Paul and I have created our own small clan, but for just a brief time that holiday, I felt like I was part of an extended family, sharing holiday stories, laughing, and comparing our family traits; just doing what families do. I was reminded that I did have a parent left, and it was actually a lovely and normalizing experience. However, it also served to make me sad and very aware of what I don't have.

It is hard to prematurely become the adult, as I have. Most people get to have their parents well into late adulthood, and that's a reality I have no experience with. My mother died when I was nineteen. My father hasn't been a functioning parent for more than ten years and will continue his slow decline into darkness and I will continue to experience my life as a person without parents. It is hard not to miss the comfort and support and accumulated wisdom of parents. If you have it, you don't know what it's like not to have it, until something happens to take it, like death or dementia. I make decisions on my own and direct my life without parental interference and input. I barely remember what parental interference is like, and I do miss what I don't have.

I miss having a normal life - parents to boss me around, to grow older alongside, and to enjoy family times with. I imagine other caregivers, orphans, and semi-orphans might feel like I do – a little removed from many of the family and social experiences that most people find routine. We stand, alone and unprotected by the comfort of parents, and sometimes it feels a bit raw, a bit painful. Losing parents also moves you into the front line of the battle of life, so to speak. There is no longer a comforting bulwark of people between you and death – you are next. It can make you keenly aware of your own mortality and of what you have and haven't done with your life – not unlike a mid-life crisis – which can cause its own sort of grief.

Once you lose one parent, you enter a territory inhabited only by those who have also lost a parent. Friends and family members will never fully understand your loss, or be able to truly enter that territory, until the same thing happens to them. You may notice a new distance between you and those people. You may find that you gravitate towards those friends and acquaintances who have citizenship in that place because they know the language and the lay of the land. Losing the other parent moves you even further still into that country, so that you are fully, if reluctantly, a citizen.

I am only forty-three and I realized that I've been half an orphan for over half my life. The only thing left to be is an orphan in name as well as in feeling and I wonder if I will feel any differently? We will all, eventually, become orphans since our parents usually die before we do, and it is important to acknowledge and feel the grief of that loss - whether one has lost parents at a young age, in middle, or old age.

*

Some caregivers experience guilt at the death of their loved one. While guilt at the death of a loved one is not unique, a caregiver's guilt can be especially multi-faceted. A caregiver can feel guilty about not doing enough or caring well enough for the care-taker; or not being with them when they died; or feeling revulsion at the dying process; or feelings of gladness that the demands are done with and the loved one is out of pain. There has probably been some resentment felt all along, so caregivers may feel remorse about that as well.

In addition, caregivers may feel that they have lost an established and well-understood role. Their schedule, duties, and responsibilities were well-defined and largely unchanging and they were focused on the goal of keeping their care receiver well and happy. Caregiving is a profession with emotional ramifications. Now, duties done and responsibilities over, what are they for? What will they do? Extra support for caregivers in this particular area is essential.

One doesn't have to be a caregiver to feel grief at the loss of one's role. We all play a role in other's lives and they play a role in ours. To lose the certainty of that can be as difficult as the physical loss of a loved one. It is important to realize that grief has many different facets, and takes many forms. People will experience loss in different ways; mourning something, for example, that might never occur to you to miss, or acting in ways you find strange. It is never appropriate to comment on how another person grieves and whether they are doing it "right" or not, because there is no "right"; everyone must go through the process in their own way. Unfortunately, friends, co-workers, and other family members may sometimes try to hurry the grieving individual through the process – either out of their own discomfort or because they have never experienced grief before and don't understand its difficulties.

Many still expect bereaved individuals to "get over" their intense feelings within months, if not weeks. Most places of employment offer a few days of grief leave, when the actual process of grieving may take up to a year or more. I'm not suggesting people deserve a year's leave from work, but I am suggesting that a few days is not enough to know to what extent your bereavement is affecting you. I would submit that a few weeks of grief leave would be more cost effective in terms of lost production and confusion and mistakes at work.

As a bereavement counselor, I have called grieving family members every month as a measured way to provide support and comfort. I now work for a hospice organization that provides bereavement services, like phone calls, for fifteen months, as a way to emphasize the continuity of care for the family. On my own, I formed the practice of sending a card or making a phone call to friends who had suffered a loss on the anniversary of that loss. All of these are ways to keep the grieving within a structure of support that acknowledges the loss and the accompanying grief.

We are trained that different cultures may experience and process grief differently than Americans. It is important that we are aware of these differences so that we don't impose our ideas of appropriate grief and grieving on others. In Chinese culture, it is considered unhealthy to talk about one's emotions, whereas in America, we are more accustomed to sharing our emotional state. In some cultures, the name of the dead person is not spoken so as not to distract them from their journey.

In the Jewish faith, for example, family members have the option of several rituals to ease the pain of bereavement and loss, including sitting Shiva, and saying Kaddish- each of which are rituals designed to pray for and honor the dead and provide comfort and closure for the living. The yahrzeit, or anniversary of the death, is a time to commemorate the loved one, including visiting the cemetery, and laying stones on top of the gravestone.

In some Native American societies, the deceased are not mentioned by name. Photographs and conversation about the person who has passed are considered inappropriate. Instead, tribes honor the dead non-verbally. Mexican-Americans celebrate the Days of the Dead, Dias de los Muertos. They believe that during this time, October 31 through November 2, the deceased can visit living relatives and friends, and families welcome their dead loved ones with feasting and celebration. Mexican culture portrays this aspect of society through art, cooking and crafts.

At Japanese-American funerals or memorial services, co-workers are expected to give a monetary gift in an envelope to the family. Called a "koden," the amount is based on the type of gift you may have received from the deceased or the family in similar circumstances. Different Buddhist sects carry out different rituals at different times.

In general, the first seven days after death are the most important for the grieving rituals. The mourners say prayers and practice meditation that will help the decreased achieve the transformation into rebirth. This continues for 49 days. The eldest son selects and decorates the altar for use in the funeral service. After the cremation of the body, those who attended the funeral service receive food and gifts.

At Buddhist funerals, the family members appreciate gifts of vegetarian food. The family will usually host an incense ceremony, but guests may observe only and do not need to participate. At Islamic funerals, women dress modestly, covering their heads and arms. On some occasions, only men can attend the burial service.

Chinese tradition holds that the soul lives on after death, and that the spirit of the deceased will return to his home seven days after death. The family is expected to remain in each of their rooms, and a red plaque is placed over the main entrance to show the spirit the way home. Flour or rice is scattered on the floor, so that when the loved one returns home, he will be able to see his footprints.

Family members are expected to burn paper representing money and other material possessions for the departed after death. Family members also burn this paper during the annual day of memory in April, when they visit the graves of relatives. The money is for the deceased to use in the afterlife.

Unfortunately, most of us who aren't part of a specific ethnic or religious group don't have many set procedures or rituals to help us navigate the bereavement process – or, for that matter, some of the other significant life stages. Rituals can serve, not only to mark these occasions, but also to comfort and provide guidance through the transitions they represent.

There are practices and procedures that provide healthy, constructive, and supportive methods of dying and grieving. Perhaps we could follow the examples of other cultures, ethnic or religious bodies that still maintain ritual structures, to find ways to better experience, and process, our grief and loss. Rituals like lighting candles at certain times of day and thinking of lost loved ones; doing an activity or making a meal a loved one enjoyed. There are healthy ways to continue to incorporate a lost loved one into present-day life.

*

I have heard it said that grief never truly goes away, we just become more adept at coping with it. I believe that this is true. We never truly heal from grief, we just learn to live with it. I still miss my mother every day, and it's been twenty-five years since she died. I grieve my father every day and he hasn't even died yet. Sometimes it seems as if I have experience with almost every kind of grief there is – chronic illness, the final grief of a parent's death, the death of friends and family members, the drama and sadness of divorce, and the ambiguous grief of losing someone to dementia. I am steeped in grief, like a teabag left too long in the cup.

I have found that doing hospice work and bereavement counseling has made me more comfortable with the realities of death and loss and grief. It has been an honor and an education to be present at the deaths of others, and to witness, and, hopefully, help ease the ensuing grief. We will all, at some point, suffer a loss of a loved one and the accompanying grief – there is no avoiding it. I think that the more we talk about it, normalize it, allow ourselves to experience it, and bring it back into our family lives, the less it will exist as an alarming, mysterious, and negative experience.

A Few Things I Figured Out.

- We must make sure we allow ourselves to grieve, and whatever way we do it is exactly right. Be aware of social expectations and fears around grief – it is a natural, human, acceptable response to loss. It can manifest in multiple different ways, both physical and emotional. Don't let anyone decide what a normal grieving process is for you. Take the time for self-care and feeling your loss. Try not to make any big decisions. If you do feel that normal grieving has tipped over into serious depression and lack of function, get help from a physician or licensed therapist. You don't have to suffer. Many local hospice organizations and hospitals now offer bereavement counseling and support groups. Locate one in your area. There is no shame in admitting that you need a little extra help and support during this time.
- Loss of a parent can be a difficult experience with its own special stresses and consequences. It can be hard to lose the comfort and support provided by parents, as well as the

grounding and the history they hold for us. Finding a support group specific to parental loss is a good idea since friends who haven't experienced similar may not understand.

- Accept that there may be feelings of resentment, guilt, and remorse around your loved one's death, especially if you were their caregiver. Be aware of feelings of inadequacy or that you didn't do enough. You may have to grieve the loss of your role as a caregiver, as well.

- None of us would wish ambiguous loss on anyone, but if one is in it, the important thing is to be aware of it. Be aware of unexpected and unexplained depression and anxiety. Allow yourself to feel the utter sadness and unfairness of the situation, just as if your loved one had actually died. Use anticipatory grief as another tool in your tool belt, one that will help you let go of your loved one in a kinder and gentler manner, rather than letting it work against you. People who have mentally lost a loved one who is still physically alive, have the right to grieve just as much as those who are suffering from the actual death of a loved one. This can be a difficult concept to explain to others. Most people are much better at understanding the grief of a finished loss. It can be harder for them to comprehend and accept that the process might be going on for a long time, and that you might need their help and patience for that length of time.

- Develop your own rituals to honor your loved one and your grief at their loss. Light candles in their memory, make favorite foods, make an altar of special items and pictures, visit places that were special. All of these are ways of making space for our legitimate feelings and the memory of a person who was special to us. Grieve the loss of their role in your life as well as your role in theirs.

23.

Final Destination.

"T'is time to be old, To take in sail: The gods of bounds, Who sets to seas a shore, Came to me in his fatal rounds, And said: 'No more!" Ralph Waldo Emerson

At first, I saw nothing out of the ordinary. The little white note card closely resembled all the other little white cards fluttering like dusty, forgotten butterfly wings pinned against a board. This particular card was taped haphazardly on the inside of the cupboard door, among notes, fast food receipts, calendar pages, and reminders comprising a collage of events and thoughts. My name, written in big letters on the nondescript card, caught my eye. I didn't have time to look at it too closely, before Dad approached.

His eyes sharpened as he took in the details of my face, striving to make connections in his tattered brain. Old age and illness had softened what once seemed immutable, unchanging. It had seemed to me that my father would remain strong and true forever, like a tree rooted in the forest floor. Now, shorter and slightly bent over, eyes foggy and uncertain, his muscles and skin had slackened, helping the disease steal expression from his face. As I moved closer to hug him, my nose caught the faint cologne of dementia; long-ago meals, age, and seldom-washed underwear.

Dad shuffled off to his bathroom to prepare for our journey to lunch. I waited patiently until sure he had closed the door since he still got a little snippy if he thought I was prying through his things or trying to find his checkbook. I wanted a closer look at the piece of paper that had attracted my attention. Under my name he had written in capital letters in the controlled, block printing he'd learned as an engineering student, "My Epitah." The name Waldo-Emerson was written underneath, followed by four lines of a poem I did not recognize.

Familiar, of course, with the name Ralph Waldo Emerson, I had little real knowledge of his actual work. However, the beauty of the words shone clearly through the smudged Bic pen ink and they moved me. Evidently, at some point Dad had read or seen the poem and been touched by it as well. I extrapolated from the misspelled heading that he wanted it to be used as his epitaph.

I was just generally surprised that my father might have any knowledge of something like this. Not a man given to poetry, or even many words, my father had a rigid sense of duty and an ascetic's views of pleasure. He rarely gave himself respite from work, only occasionally indulging in things that diverted or entertained him. Though he was an extremely intelligent man, I rarely saw him read a book. I never saw him with any books of poetry, never thought to even associate him with such a thing.

Did he find and become familiar with this arrangement of words years ago? Or had he merely seen the poem at some point and felt it strike a chord deep within him - enough so that he remembered it even as other memories had been wiped clean from his mind. When had he written this card? I had never seen it before but that didn't mean anything – it could have been among his clutter of papers for years, or he may have just written it.

As I heard the rattle of the doorknob signifying Dad's exit from the bathroom, I quickly nudged the cupboard door shut and took a giant sideways step back to the place I was standing when he left. Unfortunately, I didn't have enough time to grab the card and hide it in my jacket. After we had lunch, I dropped him off and continued to muse on my discovery well into my long drive home.

I adore words and am never happier than when I see a well-crafted or lyrical sentence. I have a good memory, and words and phrases tend to stick in my head. I couldn't remember all of the words in the verses I'd seen and many of them were misspelled or fragmented but I recalled enough to be struck by their simple beauty. For days afterward, I pondered on the entire scene. I found my mind focusing over and over on the different elements contained within that 3x5 card. I was surprised that he had even given any thought to his epitaph. This was a man who had had no financial or medical plan at all, who had not even written out a will, let alone a carefully planned and documented funeral plan!

Even more to the point, his religion denied the very existence of disease or death. Dad was a Christian Scientist, a belief system in which there exists no illness, dysfunction, or death. These are thought to be manifestations of evil, error, incorrect thought, and firmly kept out of mind. There are no funerals within the Church. Members who die simply vanish and are rarely spoken of again.

The paper did remind me of a conversation that took place during one of our long summer walks by the lake. He asked me what I thought about death and what kind of arrangements I wanted made after I died. Surprised that he would talk about death, I told him what I thought about it all, and about my plans to be cremated. Taking courage from his seeming willingness to talk about a formerly taboo subject, I asked him what HE thought, and what he wanted done after his death. He stated very clearly that he wanted to be cremated, his ashes spread over the lakefront property that we had owned for forty years, where he had spent so much of his time swimming and watching the ducks.

I agreed that this sounded very nice, and promised I would take care of it when the time came. We were even able to briefly discuss what it would mean to be on life support, and the fact that we agreed that neither one of us would want to live that way. We had a really lovely, if surprising, discussion; one that stands out for me as a highlight of our time together. I'm grateful for that conversation, not only because of the fellowship we shared that day, but also because it gave me some clue about what he wanted after his death, something I wouldn't otherwise have known. If he had been possessed of all his faculties, I sincerely doubt that we would have been talking about the subject at all.

The very fact that he had directed this missive to me and not to other caregivers – had not, in fact, written my older sister's name in wavering block letters on the white paper - made me quietly happy. Obviously, he had thought of me during the creation of the note because my name was on it. I hoped it was because of trust engendered during our caregiving journey together. I wondered at what point it had occurred to him that he might want an epitaph, or that he might have to arrange one for himself?

What thought or event had sparked the action of finding the poem, finding the card, and laboriously writing it all down with what little remained to him of comprehension and the ability to write?

What had been going through his mind at the time, and why hadn't he spoken of it to me? So every time I visited Dad in the weeks after, I looked for the card, but couldn't find it, until finally, one afternoon, it resurfaced. Taking no chances this time, I snatched it from where it hung lopsidedly and tucked it away in my purse.

From the few words that Dad had been able to write on the card, I was able to track down the piece on the Internet. The poem turned out to be both lovely and evocative, employing as it did images of the sea and sailing to represent death and dying, and an elusive and wind-tossed God who rests among the elements of the world. It perfectly reflected those few things that had given Dad so much pleasure during his life; the sailing and swimming and relationship with the water that he had enjoyed so very much. I printed it out to keep on my desk next to the battered, misspelled little notecard.

Surprisingly, over the next few days I began to see the poem everywhere, reflecting some strange synchronicity. I found it in an Internet article celebrating the life of a well-known man, and the next day in a book I had just started reading about Alzheimer's disease. Unknowingly, Dad had picked a poem perfectly reflective of his fate. I have since learned that Emerson wrote this while suffering from the beginnings of dementia himself, probably Alzheimer's, something he'd already come to realize in 1866, when the poem was probably composed. Knowing this only raises more questions for me.

Did my dad know this when he read the poem and picked it to be his epitaph? Did he know that Emerson was most likely describing his own experiences of feeling parts of his mind and experience vanish? Or did its images of the sea and nature just appeal to him and his love of boating and water? What was it, exactly, that moved my father to look through the mistiness of his mind, remember this poem, and jot it down on a card with my name on it?

Like many other things about my father, these are questions to which I will never know the answer, both because the card came to me too late in my father's disease, and because we were not accustomed to having conversations of this nature with each other – which is a loss for both of us, I think. All I have about his feelings and ideas around his death is this little card and that short conversation we had years ago.

*

I've told this story because it encompasses so perfectly for me the ways we communicate, or don't communicate, with our loved ones about how we, and they, want the end of their lives to look. Most people when asked say that they would like a "good death," which is a subjective concept and specific to each individual. Most people would probably agree that it means lucidity up to the end; closure of emotional and personal issues and desires; limited pain, discomfort, and mess, and often the loving presence of family. Unfortunately, few have discussed it with the individuals who will probably be facilitating it.

Experts have come up with the phrase, "end of life", as a comprehensive way to describe all of those events, issues, and procedures that happen as an individual reaches death. Issues such as: who do you want to be with you as you die; *where* do you want to be, at home or in a hospital; do you want serious medical intervention, or a peaceful death; and what do you want done after your death? After all, there is much more to death than simply death.

As caregivers, we will probably face the final journey with our loved one. Many of you may already have done so. As a caregiver and caregiver advocate, I understand that there is generally only one way that caregiving ends - someday, perhaps sooner rather than later, my father will die. At some point, after many years of care, or maybe only a few; after struggles and challenges; after illness and doctor's visits and palliative care – the suffering always comes to an end. Our care receiver is free, as are we, their caregivers, and everything changes again. As sad and shocking as it can sometimes feel – all life ends. Just before that happens, though, there are things that need to be done, and decided, and discussed.

In the past, most people died at home in the presence of their family, sustaining the belief that death was a natural part of life. In the past, children were aware of aging and death because they witnessed these processes happening to their grandparents. They most likely were also involved in care to a certain extent, with the supervision and assistance of a parent. Somehow, that frank acceptance of a natural process has gotten lost. People don't experience death regularly and don't want to think or talk about it.

I have a fair amount of experience with aging and end-of-life issues; enough so that when an individual asks me how and when to start conversations with a family about the end of life, I start answering before they've even finished the question. Now is the time to start the discussion. <u>Now</u> is the time to begin discussing things like important healthcare and end-of-life wishes, finances, housing, where important documents are kept, and what final arrangements have been made. Begin now because you may have to have more than one discussion before any concrete decisions or plans will be made, and you may have less lucid time with that person than you think.

Obviously, my own family was not the type to have these conversations. For instance, most of our relatives had no idea my mother was dying until after she died because she didn't <u>want</u> us to tell them. She left no instructions or memorial plan, relying on my father, and, I suppose, my sibling and I, to take care of everything. I remember clearly being clueless about how to plan a memorial service; where it should take place; how you told everyone, what was said and done and in what order. And yet, I was still given the responsibility of arranging it.

And of course, my father was no better. It had to wait until he was stricken by dementia before we could even begin to talk about death and final wishes. Would I have preferred to obtain this information in the usual manner, through long talks with a lucid parent, where discussion is possible and options are mooted, and people are comforted? Of course. But I have to work with what little I have.

Nobody really wants to have these discussions, especially someone who is aging and ill – they are uncomfortable, can be contentious, and take a lot of energy. Few people want to even think about their own death, let alone make decisions. However, having these issues settled as clearly and completely as possible will ease everyone's path considerably in the future. Families can feel uncomfortable talking about the impending death of a loved one, as if they were hurrying the process along, or giving up hope, or because they think that their loved one doesn't want to talk about it. Thus, they often *don't* talk about it, leaving everyone unprepared for the experience, and the loved one alone and apprehensive about what is coming.

It has actually been my experience doing hospice care that the reverse is true: many people *want* to talk about things like their own death and their feelings about the process– especially if they are approaching the end of their life. They want to share their lives, their thoughts and fears, what they would like to be known or remembered about them, and even what their epitaphs and eulogies might be. Unfortunately, this can sometimes be difficult for friends and family to hear because it means admitting to the fact that death is imminent or gives the impression that hope is gone, so they change the subject or shut down any conversations about it.

We all realize these are painful and sad topics to discuss, but now is the time to put aside our own feelings and discomfort and act in a way that supports what the dying person needs and wants. There is no more useful purpose in guarding personal, practical information, needs or wishes. Financial and medical issues will inevitably begin to arise and it is best to have some sort of framework. The fact is that actions will need to be taken, regardless of whether information is divulged or not.

Remind your loved one that now is the chance for them to have their say about what those actions are and how they look, otherwise, they will have to be happy with *your* choices. Remember that the conversations may not proceed as you thought they might, or how the books describe. What's important is that you get the information, how you get it is irrelevant.

There are other types of conversations I would also encourage people to start having now - conversations with and about your loved one and your relationship with them. What was their life like; what do they remember most and what did they enjoy; and what are they thinking about or feeling as they approach the end. If it's comfortable for both of you, you can talk about your relationship with them.

I will very much miss these kinds of conversations people are able to have with their loved ones at the end of life. What we think of as the emotional wrap-up. I won't be able to tell my dad what he meant to me, or find out what I meant to him. I will not be able to discuss problems I have had with my father, and hear that he is sorry, and feel that I can forgive. We will not be able to discuss past events, or my mother, or what he loved or regrets most about his life. My father will die silent and already vanished; all I will have are the conversations we shared when he was still a little bit lucid.

It is entirely possible that yours was the type of family that had these conversations early and often. If that is the case, then you are to be envied - many people wish for that kind of openness and honesty in their familial relationships. If you do not belong to a family that communicated openly, now is the time to examine old patterns of communication and see if they are still relevant and helpful to the current situation.

We've all heard the cliché about not waiting until it's too late to express everything you want your loved one to know, but in this case, it's definitely something to think about. I urge the people I speak with now to really try to make the time and effort to have these conversations now.

*

Out of all of my therapeutic volunteer experiences, what I have found most rewarding is my work with hospice and bereavement support. In our culture, few of us are familiar with or well prepared for death or grief, which is often when people are at their most vulnerable and confused. We need better education as well as people and ways that can help ease this process.

This is why I think the modern hospice movement is doing such good work; bringing death and dying back into the family and back into "normal" life. In my experience, hospice care can provide families and individuals with the "good death" they might be looking for. I love being a hospice volunteer for just this reason. If I can help one person with the overwhelming feelings from the death of a loved one, then I have done good work.

The philosophy of hospice care is based on the idea of death as a natural process; it proposes to neither hasten nor postpone death's advance, but instead to manage care as well as possible until death arrives. At its simplest, hospice exists to make a dying patient comfortable, but does not seek to provide a cure or any aggressive medical treatment. Hospice provides physical, social, psychological, emotional, and spiritual solutions to the questions and problems of terminal illness.

Some people continue to view hospice with suspicion because there is still a strong perception it is involved with euthanasia or is a form of mercy killing, which couldn't be further from the truth. On the contrary, hospice does not want to enroll a patient too early, while there may still be a chance for a cure, or while there could still be some benefit from aggressive medical treatments. It is a fact that very few hospice patients come too early to hospice – most come too late, preventing them from accessing all the benefits and solace that hospice can provide.

It is designed to provide care, support and guidance - not only for the patient, but also for the patient's family and loved ones – throughout the sometimes confusing and always emotional dying process. Hospice care is fortunately a Medicare covered benefit which is one reason it can be such a helpful way for low income patients to receive necessary services. Pain, nausea, confusion, toileting, re-positioning, and bathing are just some of the tasks that hospice care performs, as well as helping families apply for benefits and make legal and funeral arrangements.

Most of all, hospice care provides an opportunity and safe space for patient, caregiver, and family to talk about difficult issues and whatever else is important and even provides grief specialists to support families for a year or more after death. In my experience, hospice care acts as an advocate for the patient and family.

I'm not sure exactly when it happened that the normal, family and community-centered experience that is dying was hijacked and made into a "morbid", medicalized, hospital-centered event: probably around the same time that giving birth became a hospital-centered event. As a society, we appear to fear death - even speaking about aging and death is considered morbid and depressing. We treat death, the most natural physical event next to birth, as a medical condition needing to be fixed, relegating our aging to hospital beds, Intensive Care Units, and life-sustaining machinery while spending millions. Death is no longer a familiar experience – it is surrounded by machines and sterility.

We need to take more responsibility for our own life, and death, decisions. Should we let doctors talk us, or our loved ones, into expensive, extensive treatments? Should we continue to medicate or agree to the use of a feeding tube, which can be very uncomfortable and invasive, when there isn't any point? If there are no other medical problems or if the problems aren't fixable, should we just leave people alone to die in the way they see fit?

I also feel, and so do many doctors, that we should we train our medical professionals more thoroughly on the dying process and ways it could be approached. Doctors were not trained in how to manage the emotional well-being and comfort of the dying and their families, although fortunately that is starting to change. I doubt that death will ever be an easy thing for people to manage or cope with, signifying as it does our mortality and that of the ones we love as well, however, openness and honesty can only improve the process for everyone. This is why I have come to believe that discussions about end of life are so important for the whole family to have, so nobody feels unsupported or under-informed and scared.

Discussing concepts like hospice and palliative care, death-with-dignity options, and a reassessment of grief and the realities and needs of former caregivers and the bereaved will allow us to step forward into the natural process that is end of life.

The more familiar and comfortable we become with end of life, the more successfully we will be able to navigate it, either to have the kind of death *we* want, or to help our loved ones to have the death *they* want – the "good death." There is no specific formula for this, since each person's wishes will be different, but it refers, in general, to a death free from pain, worry, and stress, that might possibly include family, and an emotional review of the patient's life.

*

Once the end has taken place, your loved one is gone, the confusion and effort of the memorial is over, and family has gone home: then what? What comes next can be a difficult test of endurance and patience. Unfortunately, the end of life sometimes takes a lot longer to end and is a lot more complicated than anticipated because of the emotional and practical results of death. I'm talking about bereavement, grief, bureaucracy, paperwork, and final resolution. Granted, I have not yet had to face this with Dad, and I have only the foggiest memory of what he had to manage when my mom died. I am trying to prepare for it as best I can, however, by being aware of the process and what will be required.

In the midst of grieving are the practical responsibilities of death. Things like paperwork, death certificates, closing out bank and investment accounts, cleaning out a residence, and disposing of clothes and personal affects. Some of these things can be put off a few months, although settling an estate should probably be initiated - it tends to take on a life of its own because of probate and official procedures.

Once again, try to avoid making big financial or contractual decisions until you have moved out of the worst of the grieving process. Many of those issues can wait a few months. If you can, hire an attorney and/or accountant who can help you navigate these final requirements; you can also call in favors from any friends who have this knowledge.

Cleaning out the residence, whether house, condo, assisted living apartment, or nursing home room can be a challenging and emotional experience. You may have already performed this job as your loved one downsized or money was needed for care. I, of course, have already finished this tough job, largely because I was afraid the house might fall down before I achieved it. It was an extended (6 month) process that required a great deal of time and energy and included a lot of emotional moments.

My father had hoarded a lot of material in the latter days of his illness; however, he had also been in the habit of keeping every important – and not so important – piece of paper that crossed his desk. There were at least six filing cabinets in the house, full of paper, in addition to packed banker's boxes. Many of my mother's possessions still filled the house, as well as some things from my grandparents! My father had also kept an extensive shop in the garage that took several weeks to clean out. I hired a professional – a lovely woman whose career was de-cluttering houses, organizing closets, and assisting hoarders to clean out their houses. I also had several friends who unselfishly gave their time to help me out.

In the end, we filled many, many dumpsters with trash and unwanted objects, but I also found a lot of sentimental objects and papers that I now treasure. I recommend to everyone I talk to that they need to either hire help or ask their friends for it. Cleaning out years and years of accumulated life is not easy and definitely not something to be done alone.

In one respect, my sibling and I were fortunate: we each had an idea of what objects and keepsakes we wanted and there was no arguing over a desired piece of furniture or painting. It was relatively easy to divide everything up. We held an estate sale to dispose of everything else.

*

I hope and believe that as a society we are starting to deal with end of life issues a little bit more honestly and clearly. It seems pretty clear that we need to move dying out of morbid, taboo territory and back into being a natural, accepted part of family life. The growth of hospice and palliative care gives me hope that we can all experience the death we would most want. There are still too many complications in terms of the medical community, the curative goals of physicians, and the tendency to keep people alive long after what is natural and humane. I hope that we can continue to open the conversation into these issues.

I definitely plan to enroll my dad in a hospice program at the appropriate time, because I want him to have all the care, comfort, and support to which he is entitled. I also know that *I* will need as much comfort and support as I can get as his end approaches – knowing what I know of hospice care only makes me more confident that they will be able to help the both of us. Until that time, I am so grateful that I have dad under the radar, so to speak, when it comes to the medical sphere.

He has a doctor that visits him in his home regularly, but since Dad has no real medical issues (other than dementia), there is no reason for him to need much medical care or many medications. Unlike many people his age, he is only on some vitamins and an anti-depressant. I plan to manage the end of his life the way I imagine he would have, as a Christian Scientist, with limited medical intervention. I imagine – and hope - that I will be able to keep him in his home as he drifts away – calling in hospice care when the time is right – and hope to avoid the hassle, confusion, and heartbreak of being in the hospital.

We can no longer talk about it, but I hope to give him the good death he may have wanted. I hope that I am able to help him die in the most comfortable, painless, dignified way possible, in just the way I imagine he might have wanted. I am touched by his last message to me, and I will be faithful about making it his epitaph.

A Few Things I Figured Out.

- Although I realize that end of life issues have inescapable emotional baggage, the more they can be dealt with as straightforward, business-like, practical decisions, the better off everyone will be in the future. Initiate the end of life conversation, repeatedly if necessary. Even if your family can't quite keep it business-like, at least some information will be exchanged. Keep having the conversations and hopefully, things will get easier. Ask a lawyer, pastor, or trusted friend to help mediate if the conversation breaks down.

- Make sure you are creating the space and time to encourage conversations about end of life care like hospice and palliative care, extreme medical interventions, and where and how the care-taker would prefer to end their days. Try to speak about dying, memorials, funerals, and any wishes after death. Discuss what a "good death" means for that person. It will be too late to discuss these things after dementia and illness have stolen words and wishes, thoughts and dreams - and it will certainly be too late after death. Have the conversations that you've always wanted to have, be with the person in the way you've always wanted to be – now is the time, right where you are is the place.

- Like the note card exchange my father and I had, conversations about end of life may not resemble what you are expecting or have been told is correct. Listen and pay attention to what is being said and done, or not said, as the case may be. Extrapolate what you can from the information you glean, go with what you know of that person, and with your gut.

- The more prepared one is for the practical details of what is to come - whether it is deciding who will care for the patient, knowing what the end of life will look like, or what kind of service to have – the less stressed one will be. Is there a financial framework in place for paying bills and hiring care, and, if so, what are the details? Is there one person empowered to make financial and healthcare decisions and has the official paperwork been done to ensure this? What are the healthcare wishes of the care-taker and what kind of medical interventions do they authorize? Is there a Will, and where is it? What are the end of life care wishes of the care-taker, like hospice care, and what would they like done after their death in terms of services and burial?

- The processes at the end of a life are complex and challenging. If possible, get professional help with the legal and financial responsibilities. Cleaning out a family home can be a difficult emotional process. Siblings may argue over time spent, or objects wanted, or anything at all. If possible, go through furniture and precious objects in advance with everyone involved – marking which item goes to which person. Give yourself time, if possible, to perform this task without stress and time restraints. Give yourself permission to feel all the feelings that will come up from it.

24.

What The Future Holds.

"There are only four kinds of people in the world - those who have been caregivers, those who currently are caregivers, those who will be caregivers, and those who will need caregivers." Rosalynn Carter

The first recorded use of the term "caregiving" was in 1975, according to Merriam-Webster's Collegiate Dictionary. A family caregiver is defined as, "A person who cares for someone who is sick or disabled." The British organization, Carers UK, provides a more detailed and specific description; "People who provide unpaid care by looking after an ill, frail, or disabled family member, friend, or partner." One individual providing care to another, out of love, duty, or familial obligation, usually without remuneration.

No matter what you call it, caregiving is a job, and it is a tough one - without pay, official benefits, vacation or sick time, or, quite often, co-workers to help share the load. Caregiving requires, among other things: the patience and diversionary skills of an elementary school teacher; advanced nursing skills, pharmaceutical knowledge, and diagnostic abilities; nutritional knowledge and advanced cooking capabilities; occupational skills and problem-solving abilities; and the patience and compassion of Mother Theresa.

Unfortunately, although "family," caregiving represents an extensive economic savings to the government, it is still regarded as a family issue; a role that people will fulfill out of love or duty, without pay, benefits, or much public or societal support or understanding. Caregiving and everything that is required from modern-day caregivers has changed drastically, while society and the government are struggling to catch up to, and deal with, these new realities. Caregivers need money and they support.

The need for caregiving is definitely growing. It is not a passing phenomenon. It is not a brief statistical uptick. The horse has left the barn, and there's no point in closing the door. Everywhere I go, I run into people who have been touched in some way by aging, dementia, or a loved one's need for care – whether it's a parent, a grandparent, a spouse, or a friend. A few years ago, for an entire summer, from Hawaii to Chicago, I heard stories about parents in denial, dementia diagnoses', missing-in-action family members, nursing home nightmares, financial struggles, plans for memorial services. It is no longer the experience of a friend of someone we know, it is now our experience.

*

Here are some important statistics. 13% of the American population is sixty-five and over; it will be closer to 20% by 2030. The number of people over age 85 will jump from 5.7 million to 19 million by 2050. There are an estimated 44.4 million American caregivers who provide unpaid care to an adult age 18 or older, in an estimated 22.9 million households. Nearly half of all caregivers say they provide eight hours of care per week and one in five say they provide more than 40 hours of care per week.

One study revealed that persons with Alzheimer's disease required an average of 70 hours of care per week, with 62 of those hours provided by a primary caregiver. The great majority of caregivers are helping relatives. The average length of caregiving is 4.3 years. Caregivers tend to live near the people they care for, but not always, which increases the difficulty of the job.

Among caregivers who do not live with the person they care for, a large majority say they live within an hour of their care recipient and 74% say they visit at least once a week. One in four says the person they care for lives with them. Many caregivers fulfill multiple roles since most are married or living with a partner and most work while managing caregiving responsibilities at the same time. Women make up 80% of the caregivers in our nation.

More than one in three caregivers say no one else provided unpaid help to the person they care for during the past twelve months. Using the services of paid personal helpers is less common than obtaining help from unpaid caregivers. Among caregivers who help those living outside of a nursing home, only four in ten say their care recipient received paid services from an aide or nurse, hired housekeeper, or other people who are paid to help the care recipient during the past twelve months.

Almost half of caregivers say they need help managing their stress and finding time for themselves. They are also more likely to say that they have less time for friends and family, as well as vacations, hobbies or their own social activities. Nearly half of caregivers say they are getting less exercise than before becoming a caregiver. Caregivers perceive their own health status to be lower than that of their care receiver. One in eight caregivers will become injured as a result of caregiving. According to the American

Academy of Family Physicians, depression is the most common health problem among family caregivers.

What seems to be definite is that the crisis around dementia, caregiving, aging, and healthcare is getting worse. Demands on individual, family, and governmental resources are only going to grow. Aging, in general, and dementia, in particular, are about to become an oceanic undertow that will pull us under as a society if actions are not taken.

An estimated 5.3 million people in the US suffer from Alzheimer's and 1.3 million suffer from Lewy body dementia – and that's just the two most common dementia syndromes. Early-onset dementia is on the rise, as well, affecting more and more people under the age of 65.

By 2009, more than 61.6 million people in the U.S. provided unpaid care at a value of 450 billion. And yet, family caregivers are crumbling under the stress of doing it all. Families are becoming destitute and dysfunctional, trying to provide care. Our society and our government refuses to believe the fact that our social, medical, and financial structures are entirely insufficient for what is coming. We must face the fact that a large part of our population is aging; the Baby Boom Generation is heading into old age at a rapid rate, and our technology has allowed us to extend life much further than ever before. We are already unable to meet the financial, physical, and emotional needs of the aging and ill we currently have, without adding more.

Unfortunately, it can be difficult to move society into exploring, attempting to understand, and taking action against that which scares us. It can be even more difficult to convince those in power to spend the money necessary to address the problem. Instead, we remain close-minded which can actually hinder progress in the care and assistance of those who need it most - in other words, the aging, the ill, and their caregivers. This short-sighted attitude is already preventing caregivers and dementia sufferers from getting the benefits and support they need. There never seems to be enough time, money, or support and caregivers are bearing the brunt of the demands of care.

Old financial, medical, social, and governmental systems will only hamper efforts to address the coming problems of an aging population. Medicaid is very difficult to obtain, and requires an individual to spend down their assets almost completely before granting aid – taking away everything that person may have spent their life building. Medicare, designed for the aging, pays for some health care and hospitalization, but insists on seeing visible, quantifiable improvement when paying for skilled nursing; and it doesn't cover long-term care at all, the one thing that most families need.

Other countries are beginning to react to this burgeoning problem by taking a more enlightened view on the job of caregivers. France allows six months of unpaid leave and recently passed a bill giving government payments to caregivers for 3 weeks, at $62 a day. In Scotland, caregivers are viewed as partners in the provision of care. Support services, including those meeting medical and emotional needs, are provided to caregivers are regarded as part of the dependent's package of care. In other words, caregivers in Scotland are vital, and paid, members of the dependent's health care.

Carers in Australia save the government over $30 billion a year and are starting to be awarded the benefits and respect they deserve. Although the US government passed the Family Leave Act a few years ago, mandating that employers provide an employee several weeks of unpaid leave in case of a family emergency, it doesn't go far enough to support caregivers. Unpaid leave is good, but paid leave would be better.

*

There's a saying that if you've met one person with dementia – you've met one person with dementia. In essence, the disease is so complex that no one symptom or sign or behavior defines it – it doesn't follow one path, or look the same way twice. The same could be said about the undertaking that is caregiving: one person giving care will have a totally different experience than another.

Caregiving is a complex undertaking and can be many different things to different people. It involves vastly disparate requirements, experiences, and emotional states. It spawns many new realities – financial, emotional, familial, physical, and mental – many of which are rarely discussed, out of ignorance, inhibition, or insensibility.

Although the generalities of caregiving remain the same in all situations – a caregiver and a care receiver, an illness, physical and emotional challenges, and expenditure of money, time and energy – the specifics conform to no real pattern or normalcy. I think anyone whose life in any way already involves caregiving can attest to the fact that at no time is there ever anything approaching usual, typical, or regular, and in no way are conventions conformed to. Giving care is the original wild card; you can't pin it down, regulate it, or predict it, and every day will be different from the day before.

Caregiving by its very nature is a construct of dichotomies. There are two, and sometimes more, individuals, coexisting, experiencing life together yet separately - feelings, goals, and needs diverging and made more difficult by the growing gulf created by illness. Caregiving is about holding oneself accountable and feeling powerless. It is about action and reaction and growth mixed with stasis and decay. It is too often about self-worth and inferiority, guilt and relief, shame and pride.

There can be simultaneous moments of intense happiness and inconsolable despair, milestones of personal development and physical and mental disintegration, stretches of stagnation followed by transfiguration and transformation. Giving care heightens, magnifies, and redefines the elements that already make up life. It is ever-evolving and transformative, and can be, simultaneously, both the best and worst experiences of our lives; it is a double-edge sword in that it takes away as much as it gives.

Caregivers still too often operate within a peculiar cone of silence – they are a hidden, sometimes voiceless, population and I want to give them, and caregiving itself, a voice to put into words what it looks and feels like, and what it requires. My goal with this book is hopefully to make caregiving personal, both through my experiences and those of others - to tell mainstream society exactly what is going on and exactly what caregivers are facing. My goal is also to show people who are hovering on the brink of being a caregiver what they can expect, what to look out for, and how to start the process in a more healthy and effective way than I did. And finally, I want to help current caregivers feel like they have a voice – and can have a life outside of caregiving.

I hope having a discussion about the real personal, emotional, familial, and professional ramifications of being a caregiver can be helpful and bring some change. They are issues that many caregivers might wrestle with, and because of the sheer growth in numbers of caregivers now and in the future, it seems like an important subject to talk about it and make part of our dialogue. We don't really understand how deeply we as a society are indebted to family caregivers. After all, if all unpaid family caregivers were to rise up at once and refuse to work without pay and benefits from their respective governmental programs, the costs to the public would be staggering.

I want to talk about what it means to be a caregiver, attempting to live a full life alongside the diminishing life of another, and how change and growth can still come. I want to speak to caregivers like myself – younger, still going through these rites of passage and life transitions – or with the potential to go through them – to show that it's all still possible. I want to begin to transform how we think about our lives, our families, our feelings and our bodies, and how to deal with the challenging things that happen to us.

Some life events, such as caregiving, are so huge and require so much of an individual that it can be difficult for caregivers to realize that they are still leading their own lives, with all the attendant growth, transformation, relationships, and experiences. I know intimately that it can feel as if there is no hope of anything else; all dreams, goals, hopes, and loves of are no longer possible. I still maintain, however, that there can be hope – even when one is giving care.

Becoming a writer, sharing my experiences with others, and sending thoughts and feelings out into the world, to be accepted and enjoyed, has been transformative. I hope that at some point, my musings and blogging and remembering have been helpful to other caregivers. I'm certainly grateful to everyone who has read my blog over the years and even bought my book! I hope this one is even better than the first one – that it covers more things, or talks about more important issues, or is just more fun to read.

Talking to and helping other caregivers has been enormously fulfilling, by seeing how compassionate and caring people can be, and how they soldier on through the most difficult experience with courage and humor. Learning more about the end of life process and how to help families through it has given me great rewards, and being present for bereaved people, both in support groups and individual session, has taught me a great deal.

Having a core group of wonderful friends who helped me along the way has also been important, not to mention the distractions of two serious relationships with different men – one who shared the first part of my journey with Dad but turned out to be mentally ill, and one who is sharing the second part of my journey and who I ended up marrying in a beautiful ceremony when I was forty.

I have learned that it is never too late to make a change in your life. I have also learned – begrudgingly, irritatedly, and repeatedly – that every part of my life is affected by Dad's needs and my duties as a caregiver. Every part. I can't move, date, travel, work, or sleep without first thinking about how it affects my care of, and responsibility for, Dad. However, as I have made this journey with him, I have also been forced to admit that, while I have had to deal with many adverse changes and many roadblocks to a normal life, I have received rewards I could not have expected. I have continued to experience life's milestones, both because of, and in spite of, being a caregiver. It is important to remember that good things can still happen even though life is full of caregiving. That growth is still possible, even in the face of difficulty, sacrifice, and grief. I know, because it has happened to me, and because it continues to happen.

My own caregiving experience hasn't ended yet - Dad continues to drift slowly onward into infirmity and death. I do ponder what the end will look like. I think about how it feels to be an "orphan", the quiet ways my father and I talked about his wishes around death, and how it feels to get older and have all protective parental layers between you and death removed, so that you are next in line. I have made my plans for Dad's death and the immediate requirements, and I have experienced my grieving all along, however, I imagine it will still be difficult when all the final t's are crossed and i's dotted and I'm not responsible for his life any longer. Like all caregivers, I need to think about what I'll do after that.

It might go a little more slowly or not look quite like you expected, but it can still happen. You have to find a way that works for you – your own path to what you want. Or, you can compromise and make a new plan that isn't what you first wanted but which will fulfil you just the same. In very challenging cases, you may absolutely have no time for anything but caregiving and can only think about your life continuing after your care receiver is gone. Don't give up hope here, either. You can still be planning; you can still be thinking about what you want your life to be. If an aging, partially-disabled caregiver like me can have a life, so can you – you might just have to wait a bit.

My experiences and beliefs might not mirror everyone's, but I do believe that anything and everything is possible for anyone. If there is one thing I have learned, it is that, if you're open to it, if you give yourself the chance and the space, growth can come out of even the most unlikely, difficult, or horrifying situation. I do believe it is possible to continue to grow and achieve and experience life – difficult but not impossible – and absolutely necessary. If we don't grab for our own lives, no matter what it is we are going through and how much time and energy it is consuming, no one else will – we must believe that our life, and growth, matters.

If I can show even one caregiver that others recognize what they are going through, or give them hope when they are hopeless, or help them look honestly at a difficult family situation, or see something they didn't see before that might help them do their job better and live more fully - than I have succeeded. If I can help one person - whether they are already involved in caregiving, about to be involved in caregiving, or dread the day they may become involved in caregiving - understand what aging, or having dementia, or giving or receiving care means, than that is a good thing.

If Rosalyn Carter is right, we must look to the future and start preparing now for what is actually already upon us. The ranks of caregiver will be growing, and they will all benefit from some help.

Joy Walker is a writer, hospice worker and bereavement counselor and works as a professional care-manager for her Father. In 2011, she published a memoir, *Three Years and Thirteen Dumpsters: Cleaning House after Dementia*, both about being her Father's live-in caregiver, and about her experiences cleaning out the family home, filled with 40 years of living, memories, and hoarded material.

She maintains an award-winning blog about caregiving, end of life issues, Lewy body dementia, and living with chronic illness.

She is a Lewy Buddy Call Counselor and Support Group Facilitator for the Lewy body dementia Association and was recently elected to the Association's Board of Directors. She is passionate about the stress and struggle of being a caregiver and finding ways in which they can be better supported.

Walker lives with her husband in Seattle, Washington. She enjoys walking, visiting her Dad, going to movies and the theater, gardening, traveling, and spending as much time reading as possible.

30% of the proceeds from the sale of the book will be donated to the Lewy Body Dementia Association.

Bibliography

Boss, Patricia. *Ambiguous Loss: Learning to Live With Unresolved Grief.* London, England: Harvard University Press, 1999.

Koenig Coste, Joanne. *Learning to Speak Alzheimer's; A Groundbreaking Approach for Everyone Dealing with the Disease.* New York: Houghton Mifflin, 2003.

Mace, Nancy and Rabins, Peter. *The 36-Hour Day.* New York: Grand Central Publishing, 1981.

Pert, Candace. *Molecules of Emotion: The Science Behind Mind-Body Medicine.* New York: Scribner, 1997.

Cohen, Elizabeth. *The Family On Beartown Road.* New York: Random House, 2003.

Kubler-Ross, Elizabeth. *On Death and Dying.* New York: Scribner, 1997.

Maslow, Abraham. *A Theory of Human Motivation.* Psychological Review 50, 1943.

Types of Dementia

Alzheimers is characterized by loss of short-term memory leading to a denigration of all types of memory and other cognitive abilities. It leads to difficulties with executive functions: inability to perform tasks like driving, reading, caring for oneself, and, eventually, speaking, eating, and even breathing. It has become almost interchangeable with the word, "dementia," which is actually an umbrella term describing the common, progressive cognitive symptoms and neurological issues shared by several diseases. Its symptoms are well known and reported and its treatments are fairly straightforward. It is the most common cause of dementia, affecting around five million people in the US.

Alzheimer's disease, first described by the German neurologist Alois Alzheimer, is a physical disease affecting the brain. During the course of the disease, protein "plaques" and "tangles" develop in the structure of the brain, leading to the death of brain cells. People with Alzheimer's also have a shortage of some important chemicals in their brain. These chemicals are involved with the transmission of messages within the brain. Alzheimer's is a progressive disease, which means that gradually, over time, more parts of the brain are damaged. As this happens, the symptoms become more severe.

People in the early stages of Alzheimer's disease may experience lapses of memory and have problems finding the right words. As the disease progresses, they may become confused and forget names of people and places, and appointments and recent events. They may feel frustrated by their symptoms, experience mood swings, and become more withdrawn and isolated. They may have difficulty carrying out everyday activities like cooking, dressing, shopping, and paying bills. As the disease progresses, people with Alzheimer's will need more support from those who care for them. Eventually, they will need help with all their daily activities.

While there are some common symptoms of Alzheimer's disease, it is important to remember that everyone is unique. No two people are likely to experience Alzheimer's disease in the same way. Recently, some doctors have begun to use the term mild cognitive impairment (MCI) when an individual has difficulty remembering things or thinking clearly but the symptoms are not severe enough to warrant a diagnosis of Alzheimer's disease. Recent research has shown that individuals with MCI have an increased risk of developing Alzheimer's disease.

Frontotemporal dementia is one of the less common forms of dementia. The term covers a range of specific conditions. It is sometimes called Pick's disease or frontal lobe dementia. The word frontotemporal refers to the two lobes of the brain that are damaged in this form of dementia. The frontal lobes of the brain – situated behind the forehead – control behaviour and emotions, particularly on the right side of the brain. They also control language, usually on the left.

The temporal lobes – on either side of the brain – have many roles. Frontotemporal dementia is caused when nerve cells in the frontal and/or temporal lobes of the brain die and the pathways that connect them change. There is also some loss of important chemical messengers. Over time, the brain tissue in the frontal and temporal lobes shrinks.

This damage to the brain causes the typical symptoms of frontotemporal dementia, which include changes in personality and behaviour, and difficulties with language. Frontotemporal dementia occurs much less often than other forms of dementia. It affects men and women about equally. Frontotemporal dementia is most often diagnosed between the ages of 45 and 65, but it can also affect younger or older people.

In frontotemporal dementia, a variety of symptoms are caused by damage to different areas of the frontal and temporal lobes. As with most forms of dementia, the initial symptoms can be very subtle, but they slowly get worse as the disease progresses over several years.

The rate of progression of frontotemporal dementia varies greatly, from less than two years to 10 years or more. Research shows that on average, people live for about eight years after the start of symptoms. In the later stages of all forms of frontotemporal dementia, damage to the brain becomes more widespread. Symptoms are often then similar to those of the later stages of Alzheimer's disease. The person may become increasingly less interested in people and things and have limited communication. They may show restlessness or agitation, or behave aggressively. At this late stage someone may no longer recognize friends and family, and is likely to need full-time care to meet their needs.

Dementia with Lewy bodies (DLB) is a form of dementia that shares characteristics with both Alzheimer's and Parkinson's diseases. It accounts for around ten per cent of all cases of dementia in older people and tends to be under-diagnosed. Dementia with Lewy bodies is sometimes referred to by other names, including **Lewy body dementia**. These terms refer to the same disorder. Dementia with Lewy bodies appears to affect men and women equally. As with all forms of dementia, it is more prevalent in people over the age of 65. However, in certain rare cases people under 65 may develop DLB.

Lewy bodies, named after the doctor who first identified them in 1912, are tiny, spherical protein deposits found in nerve cells. Their presence in the brain disrupts the brain's normal functioning, interrupting the action of important chemical messengers, including acetylcholine and dopamine. Researchers have yet to understand fully why Lewy bodies occur in the brain and how they cause damage. Lewy bodies are also found in the brains of people with Parkinson's disease, a progressive neurological disease that affects movement. Many people who are initially diagnosed with Parkinson's disease later go on to develop a dementia that closely resembles DLB.

Dementia with Lewy bodies is a progressive disease. This means that over time the symptoms will become worse. In general, DLB progresses at about the same rate as Alzheimer's disease, typically over several years. What confuses many caregivers and physicians are the day to day differences in awareness and ability. Sufferers may be relatively high-functioning one day, and experiencing severe hallucinations the next.

Lewy body sufferers can still possess many of their memory functions and memories: any part of the brain can be affected and can begin to malfunction and lose neural connections. The relationships between thinking and acting become cut off so that a thought no longer leads to its logical action. Cognition can actually improve and then worsen on a daily basis, which leads to caregiver confusion.

They may experience problems with attention and alertness, often have spatial disorientation and experience difficulty with "executive function", which includes difficulty in planning ahead and coordinating mental activities. Although memory is often affected, it is typically less so than in Alzheimer's disease. They may also develop the symptoms of Parkinson's disease, including slowness, muscle stiffness, trembling of the limbs, a tendency to shuffle when walking, loss of facial expression, and changes in the strength and tone of the voice.

Some individuals start out with the cognitive problems and eventually develop physical symptoms resembling those of Parkinson's, like shuffling, difficulty picking up feet, balance issues, rigid muscles, and tremors. Some people start out with the Parkinson's symptoms, and develop the cognitive issues later.

Lewy body sufferers can exhibit sleep disorders, including REM sleep behavior disorder and restless leg syndrome; disorders that may manifest years before cognitive issues. Lewy body may affect the autonomic nervous system, causing issues with blood pressure; the ability to regulate body temperature; bladder and bowel control issues, including nausea; dizziness; and sexual dysfunction. Lewy body can also cause depression and apathy.

People with LBD can have severe and negative reactions to many medications, including those that are non-prescription. Check with your doctor before administering any medication, and keep a written log detailing any symptoms or reactions that might occur with new meds. There is an excellent medication glossary on the LBDA website. Traditional anti-psychotic medication, such as Haldol, is contra-indicated for Lewy body sufferers. Newer anti-psychotics, called **atypical**, can often be helpful for LBD; drugs like Seroquel and Clozaril. The dementia medication, Exelon, has been shown to be helpful for cognitive and behavioral issues.

Anti-depressants may also help an LBD patient, but again, check with the doctor. Anesthesia, even for simple operations, has been found to affect dementia sufferers and the elderly in many negative physical ways and should influence any decisions about non-emergency or elective surgical procedures.

It is also possible to suffer from a combination of different types of dementias; some brains upon autopsy show elements of Alzheimer's and LBD, for example. Those suffering from LBD tend to live two to eight years after diagnosis.

Resources

Internet

Caregiving Resources/Respite Care.

www.caregiver.org - The Family Caregiving Alliance – One of the best, most comprehensive websites, administered by an amazing organization. State by state lists of health care, caregiving, respite, housing and financial resources.

www.joyincaregiving.org

An app! http://www.helpforalzheimersfamilies.com/alzheimers-dementia-dealing/daily-companion/

www.agingcare.com

www.kccaregiver.org

www.fulllifecare.org

www.agingwashington.org

www.eldercare.gov

www.carepond.com

www.therespite.org

www.caring.com

www.caregiver.com/

www.caregiver.org/caregiver/jsp/home.jsp

www.caregiving.com

www.elderdepot.com

www.fulllifecare.org

www.nfcacares.org

www.caregivingcafe.com/

Lewy body dementia

www.lewybodydementia.org/

www.lbdtools.com

www.lewybodydementia.org/go/caregiverburden

www.apda.com

www.nia.nih.gov/alzheimers/publication/lewy-body-dementia

www.healthline.com/Lewy body dementia/Parkinson's.

www.webmd.com/mental-health/dementia-lewy-bodies

Alzheimer's.

www.alzjourney.com/

www.alzheimers.gov/

www.alzfdn.org/

www.alz.org/

Frontotemporal Dementia.

www.theaftd.org/

www.ncbi.nlm.nih.gov/pmc/articles/PMC3735339/

Vascular Dementia.

www.helpguide.org/elder/vascular_dementia.htm

www.stroke.org/site/PageServer?pagename=vad

www.stroke.org/site/PageNavigator/HOME

End of Life

www.theconversationproject.org/

www.hospicefoundation.org

www.hospicenet.org

www.houseoflightblog.com

Forums/Online Groups/Support Groups.

Memory People Facebook group – A closed group but open to caregivers and dementia sufferers, request membership from one of their Administrators.

LBDA Forums at http://lbda.org/community/forum/. You need to contact the moderator and ask for a log-in.

Look for LBD Support Groups at http://lbda.org/content/find-support.

Check other associations for groups that represent your particular dementia.

Facility Information.

www.homecareassistanceseattle.com/index.html

www.bupa.co.uk/download-guide

www.assisted-living-directory.com/

www.aplaceformom.com

www.wsrcc.org

www.nafco.org

Good Blogs.

http://cleaninghousebook.blogspot.com

http://caregivingwithpurpose.com/category/alzheimers/

http://dementiapoetry.com/

http://lifetimesthreelivingwithlbd.blogspot.com/

http://theimperfectcaregiver.wordpress.com/

http://alzheimermonologue.wordpress.com/

http://mydementedmom.com/

http://sherizeee.blogspot.com (Living in the Shadow of Alzheimer's)

http://www.earlyonset.blogspot.com/

http://momsbrain.wordpress.com/

http://www.robertssister.com

http://alzheimersdad.blogspot.com

http://www.thieflewybodydementia.com

http://goinggentleintothatgoodnight.com/

Professional Caremanagers/Organizers.

http://www.personworks.com

http://caremanager.org

Caring With a Chronic Illness.

http://www.arthritis.org

http://www.caring.com/rheumatoid-arthritis

www.lupus.org

http://www.healingwell.com/

http://www.sprebodywork.com/

Young Caregivers.

http://www.aacy.org/

Books

These are some of the best books I've found - and read - about caregiving, dementia, aging, end of life, grief, bereavement, illness, and living.

LBD

A Caregiver's Guide to Lewy Body Dementia - James and Helen Whitworth. The Lewy body dementia Bible, a must-have.

Living With Lewy's - Amy and Gerald Throop. Excellent, information-based book that covers the whole spectrum of caregiving, from diagnosis to death.

Brain and Behavior - Joseph Friedman, MD.

Living With Lewy Body Dementia – Judy Towne Jennings PT, MA.

Alzheimer's/Dementia

The 36-Hour Day - Nancy Mace. Another must-have for caregivers.

Learning to Speak Alzheimer's – Joanne Koenig Coste. Yet another must-have.

An Unintended Journey – Janet Yagoda Shagam. I really liked this one, it gave a different type of information than some others I've read.

Alzheimer's Disease and Other Dementias, The Caregiver's Complete Survival Guide – Nataly Rubenstein.

Dementia: The Journey Ahead - Susan Kiser Scarff.

Caring for Mother - Virginia Stem Owens.

Inside the Dementia Epidemic - Martha Stettinius.

Alzheimer's: A Caregiver's Guide and Sourcebook - Howard Gruetzner.

Activities to Do With Your Parent Who Has Alzheimer's Dementia – Judith Levy.

Forget Memory - Anne Davis Basting.

A Bittersweet Season - Jane Gross.

The Forgetting: Portrait of an Epidemic - David Shenk.

General Caregiving/Medical

My Mother, Your Mother - Dennis McCollough.

Knocking on Heaven's Door - Katy Butler.

Sexuality and Dementia - Douglas Wornell, MD.

The Caregiver's Guide to Compassionate Decision Making -- Viki Kind.

The Selfish Pig's Guide to Caring - Hugh Marriott.

Caregiving - Beth Witrogen McLeod.

When the Time Comes – Paula Span.

The Caregivers – Nell Lake.

The Caregiving Wife's Handbook – Diana Denholm.

You'd Better Not Die or I'll Kill You! – Jane Heller.

The Good Caregiver - Robert Kane.

End of Life/Hospice/Grief

The End of Life Handbook - David Feldman, Andrew Lasher.

Being Mortal – Atul Gawande.

When Parents Die - Rebecca Abrams.

You'll Get Over It – Virginia Ironside.

Ambiguous Loss - Pauline Boss.

The D-Word: Talking About Dying - Sue Brayne.

Dying Well - Ira Byock.

The Hospice Handbook - Larry Beresford.

Final Gifts – Maggie Callanan, Patricia Kelley.

How We Die – Sherwin Nuland.

A Grief Observed - C.S Lewis.

Miscellaneous/Life

Transitions: Making Sense of Life's Changes - William Bridges.

The Antidote – Oliver Burkeman

Scared Sick, The Role of Childhood Trauma in Adult Disease – Robin Karr Morse.

The Molecules of Emotion - Candace Pert.

God's Perfect Child: Living and Dying in the Christian Science Church - Caroline Fraser.

Keeper - Andrea Gillies.

Toll-free LBD Caregiver Link – 800.539.9767

LBD families and caregivers can connect directly on a regional basis, through the LBD Caregiver Link, featuring "Lewy Buddies." "Lewy Buddies" are experienced LBD caregivers who share their time and experience with LBD families by:

- Listening compassionately and confidentially to the challenges of LBD families and sharing their own personal experience with LBD.
- Offering emotional support.
- Referring families to additional LBDA programs and services as appropriate for their needs.

- Please leave a message and an LBDA volunteer will return your call within 24-48 hours.

Alzheimer's Association Helpline – 800-272-3900

The Alzheimer's Association's Helpline is a toll-free number that you can call 24-hours a day, 7 days a week to get information about Alzheimer's disease. Through their National office, they have the ability to serve individuals in 140 different languages by accessing translation services.

Call to speak with a trained Helpline specialist who will provide emotional support and appropriate referrals to local resources in the 23 counties served by the Association. All calls are confidential.

Alzheimer's Foundation of America – 866-232-8484

The Alzheimer's Foundation has some great information and resources, as well as a support hotline that is available 24/7 for people who need immediate assistance and advice.

www.ingramcontent.com/pod-product-compliance
Lightning Source LLC
Chambersburg PA
CBHW071709170526
45165CB00005B/1957